Estrogen:
Is It Right for You?

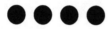

**A thorough,
factual guide
to help you
decide**

Paula Dranov

A Fireside Book · Published by Simon & Schuster
New York London Toronto Sydney Tokyo Singapore

FIRESIDE
Simon & Schuster Building
Rockefeller Center
1230 Avenue of the Americas

FIRESIDE and colophon are registered trademarks
of Simon & Schuster Inc.

DESIGNED BY BARBARA MARKS
Manufactured in the United States of America

1   3   5   7   9   10   8   6   4   2

Library of Congress Cataloging-in-Publication data
is available.

ISBN: 0-671-78130-8

1959 Height and Weight Table on page 80 courtesy
of the Metropolitan Life Insurance Company
Illustration on page 39 courtesy of The American
College of Obstetricians and Gynecologists.
Cancer of the Uterus. ACOG Patient Education
Pamphlet #AP097.
Tables on pages 67 and 68 courtesy of The National
Osteoporosis Foundation, Washington, D.C.
Table on page 93 courtesy of the American Cancer
Society

CONTENTS

Estrogen:

Is It
Right for
You?

❶❷❸

The Estrogen Question

I ALWAYS THOUGHT that estrogen replacement would be my salvation. When menopause arrived, I would simply start popping hormone pills or paste a patch to my derriere to keep my bones strong and ward off the general disintegration heralded by this momentous event. While I am generally leery of tinkering with natural chemistry, every time I looked at my mother I vowed not to let what happened to her happen to me. My mother is a beautiful woman. At eighty-eight her face is still radiant and young even though her body is crippled with Parkinson's disease. But long before the first faint tremors began, osteoporosis had left its unmistakable mark. Mother developed a dowager's hump, the spinal curvature that occurs when vertebrae crumble. Like mother, like daughter, I reasoned. Without estrogen, I was sure my bones would turn to powder. When I reached menopause, I promised myself, I would be first in line for estrogen replacement.

Then came results of a study linking estrogen replacement to an increased risk of breast cancer. Uh oh. My mother also had breast cancer. Bad study, said the experts. Not to worry. Then came another study and another. The experts began to hedge their reassurances.

The next news bulletin about estrogen replacement was much

more positive: a major study by a highly respected group of researchers confirmed what had long been suspected—estrogen replacement cuts the rate of heart disease among postmenopausal
women in half. Since more women die of heart disease than anything
else, these results made headlines.

The heart study results almost certainly will spur millions of
women toward estrogen replacement despite concerns that it may
promote breast cancer, already at epidemic levels.

In addition to the effect on heart disease, there are a number
of compelling reasons to take estrogen. The most important is its
effect on bones. Estrogen protects against osteoporosis by preventing
the bone loss that otherwise accelerates at menopause. It also can
prevent or reverse vaginal dryness (which can make sex a torture)
and the recurrent vaginal and urinary tract infections that plague
many older women. And it can extinguish hot flashes, overcome
insomnia, and, reportedly, relieve such menopausal symptoms as
irritability, memory lapses, tension, moodiness, aching joints.

Sounds terrific, but. . . .

What about estrogen and breast cancer? And uterine cancer?
Taking progestin along with estrogen seems to eliminate the additional risk of uterine cancer posed by taking estrogen alone, but
progestin itself is far from trouble free. In the first place, it brings
back your periods. But more important, it may cancel out the protection against heart disease estrogen provides.

Just what kind of chemical choreography are we being urged to
dance?

If estrogen is so safe, why does a woman need a battery of tests
before she gets her prescription? Why are only 30 percent of postmenopausal women taking it? And why do so many give it up within
a year?

If you decide to take estrogen, how long should you continue?
For the rest of your life as some doctors suggest? For five years as
others propose? What happens to your bones, your heart, and your
risk of breast cancer if you quit taking it? Why do some researchers
believe that by filling their prescriptions millions of women are
unknowingly signing up for what amounts to the most massive drug-
testing program in history? No one really knows what long-term
effects will emerge.

Statistically speaking, there is no doubt that the benefits of
estrogen replacement far outweigh the risks.

The trouble is, you can never take statistics personally. That is what this book is about. It grew out of my personal and professional curiosity as well as conversations with friends who were trying to make up their minds about estrogen replacement. As a journalist (I have been reporting and writing about health for more than twenty years) I realized that I might be able to answer many of the questions that troubled us all by pulling together as much information on the subject as I could find and by interviewing the researchers who are studying the risks and benefits of estrogen replacement.

To do this I needed to know more about what women are thinking as they approach menopause and consider estrogen replacement. How well informed are they? What deciding factors are operating? I soon realized that even though menopause no longer is the taboo topic it once was, many women are reluctant to admit that the inevitable has arrived or is fast approaching. So how was I going to find women who would own up to being the right age? The women who could not hide their age from me were my high school classmates. To their credit not one demurred when I telephoned after all these years to talk about menopause and estrogen replacement. I interviewed as many women as I could find who had considered the estrogen question. I make no claims about putting together a representative sample—my minisurvey has no scientific validity whatsoever. But it does reflect the concerns some very thoughtful women have about menopause, estrogen replacement, and the decision-making process.

If you have picked up this book, I assume that you are already taking estrogen or are nearing menopause and want to weigh the pros and cons in order to decide what to do. Let me warn you right now, the decision won't be easy. We have more than our bones to worry about. We are also getting older and facing increased risks of just about every disease there is. Heart disease is number one on that list. Breast cancer ranks near the top and, rightly or wrongly, scares many women much more than heart disease.

Given the mind-boggling array of questions about estrogen replacement and the paucity of clear-cut answers, you could just throw up your hands and say it is all too complicated and to hell with it. After all, generations of women got through menopause without estrogen. Yes they did, but they didn't live as long as we can expect to. Or maybe they didn't care that after menopause sex becomes increasingly uncomfortable. Not every woman needs estrogen to remain sexually active after menopause, but judging from what I have heard from the women I interviewed, many of us will need some kind of help.

DOES DOCTOR KNOW BEST?

In a more perfect world, our doctors would shepherd us through the twists and turns of the decision-making process, but in our world many physicians have neither the time nor the inclination to spend more than a few minutes—if that—discussing the issue. What's more, a great many physicians have very strong views on this subject and do not always recognize, much less disclose, their bias when recommending estrogen replacement or discouraging their patients from taking it. And doctors being doctors, many will happily make up your mind for you, brushing aside your questions and concerns with "doctor knows best" reassurances.

As a medical writer who has interviewed dozens of doctors, I can tell you this: clinicians—the physicians who spend most of their time treating patients rather than engaging full time in research or teaching—are very busy people. The good ones do a remarkable job of keeping abreast of medical developments. It is highly unlikely (but certainly possible) that your gynecologist or family doctor is directly engaged in research pertaining to estrogen replacement. What those practitioners know about the risks and benefits is what they read in medical journals and learn at medical meetings. Somehow, while seeing patients all day and, often, well into the night, physicians have to absorb new information, integrate it with what they already know, and then put the sum total of their knowledge into practice in treating their patients. Thrown into the mix is whatever bias they brought to the subject to start with or developed along the road.

This question of bias is a touchy one. Doctors are not purely objective men and women of science. They live in the same youth-oriented culture we do. What's more, they are heirs to a long medical tradition that views menopause as a calamity that renders women sexless, useless, and biologically and emotionally incapable of enjoying life. This attitude is no quaint artifact of the Victorian age. As recently as the 1960s (when many relatively young doctors practicing today were trained), menopause still was being described in medical literature as a tragedy.

To be fair, some of the medical pessimism may be based on experiences with women who were having a lot of trouble with menopause and on the results of studies involving women who reached menopause after hysterectomies involving the removal of their ovaries as well as uterus. The sudden loss of estrogen after this surgery brings on symptoms that are usually much more severe than those that occur when menopause arrives naturally following a long and gradual decline in estrogen levels.

Given the combined impact of a negative medical view of menopause and postmenopausal women and a cultural bias toward looking and feeling young, it is not surprising that few doctors can give us advice about menopause and estrogen untinged by their attitudes toward aging and toward women. All too often doctors buy into the preposterous and outdated stereotype of the menopausal woman as moody, cranky, rapidly wrinkling, and miserably past her prime. One of the women I interviewed, a vivacious and attractive blonde who conforms to none of the outdated notions of how menopausal women are supposed to look and feel, told me her gynecologist warned that "you'll start looking your age" when she balked at taking estrogen. This kind of "medical" thinking is a throwback to the days when estrogen was regarded as a wonder drug for women. If only it were the "youth pill" many doctors seem to think it is!

By the time you finish reading this book you will know enough about estrogen replacement to pose some tough questions to your doctor. You also will be well informed enough to evaluate the answers you get so you can make a truly informed and intelligent decision.

IS MENOPAUSE A DISEASE?

Menopause is a major health event. We stop menstruating and, all of a sudden, all sorts of things can start to go wrong with our bodies. The most immediate and startling are hot flashes and vaginal dryness. For most women, hot flashes are only temporary (although "temporary" can go on for years). The vaginal dryness is permanent and will get worse unless you do something about it.

The long-term impact of menopause, bone loss and a slow but steady increase in the rate of heart disease, is far more serious. These health risks have set off some heated medical debate on the nature of menopause. Is it, as most of us have always assumed, a change in our reproductive status signaling that we're getting older and have to be a little more vigilant about our health? Or is it, as some doctors suggest, an endocrine disease brought about by diminishing estrogen levels?

The notion that menopause could be considered a disease is pretty surprising but, upon reflection, not as far-fetched as it sounds. Wulf Utian, M.D., founder of the North American Menopause Society and chairman of the Department of Obstetrics and Gynecology at Case Western Reserve Medical School, has described menopause as a "potential endocrinopathy" (endocrine disease) that requires appropriate diagnosis and drug treatment to prevent heart disease and fractures due to osteoporosis.

Considering that, healthwise, menopause does not seem to do women a whole lot of good, regarding it as a disease may not be entirely off base. On the other hand, most women do not fall apart. Menopause and the health problems that follow may be nature's way of telling us that, in the evolutionary scheme of things, women past childbearing age are expendable. Still, we outlive men by an average of five years. A woman who reaches age fifty in the 1990s can expect to live another thirty-one years compared with twenty-six years for a man of the same age.

If menopause is a disease, then it makes sense to treat it—with estrogen, the only form of therapy effective against all the health problems associated with a dwindling supply of the estrogen our ovaries have been producing for the past forty years. But if menopause is a disease, it sure is an unusual one. Every woman, if she lives long enough, will reach menopause. But from there on the course of this "disease" is unpredictable. For some, menopausal symptoms will be severe enough to warrant treatment. If so, estrogen works much, much better than anything else available. Other women may need protection against osteoporosis. Alternatives are in the works, but, so far, estrogen is all we have. Still others will be at increasingly high risk of heart disease. Here, of course, you can reduce your risk by eating properly, exercising, and, if you smoke, giving up cigarettes.

Many women will encounter sexual difficulties that they find unacceptable. Recurrent vaginal and urinary infections are also common problems. If you are lucky, you will experience none of the above. If you are typical, you will have to reckon with one or more of these changes.

WHO NEEDS ESTROGEN?

Not even the most enthusiastic medical proponents of estrogen replacement believe every woman should take it. What we really need is a set of guidelines developed by experts in the field that we (and our doctors) could rely on to decide who needs estrogen and who doesn't. Unfortunately, the experts do not always agree on this subject. By all accounts you do not need estrogen replacement if you fall into ALL of the following categories:

• You are at low risk of osteoporosis (all women lose bone mass rapidly after menopause, but not everyone is at high risk of osteoporosis. See Chapter Five for a full discussion of this issue).

• You are not troubled by hot flashes, vaginal dryness, or other menopausal symptoms (including insomnia and joint pains).

• Your risk of heart disease is low.

• Your sex life has not suffered as a result of the physical changes that make intercourse uncomfortable and shifts in hormone balance that often throttle down the female sex drive.

You probably don't (or won't) fit neatly into all of those categories, but that is still not to say that you need estrogen replacement. And, if you feel you do, there are no rules about how long you should continue to take it. You can use it for a few months or years to relieve hot flashes or other menopausal symptoms. Or you can continue to take it indefinitely. Or you can start and stop and start again. And again.

BENEFITS VS. RISKS

Some powerful evidence suggests that long-term estrogen use will extend our lives. Researchers at the University of Southern California who followed 9000 postmenopausal women for more than seven years found that the women who took estrogen had a lower death rate than the women who did not; this difference was most striking among women who had taken estrogen for fifteen years or more: a death rate 40 percent lower than women who never took estrogen.

Impressive as those results are, much of what studies show about the benefits of estrogen replacement may be colored by the general good health of women who elect to take it. They are a fairly elitist group: most women taking estrogen today are white, affluent, slim, well educated, and health conscious. This is a profile of women who are at high risk for osteoporosis, low risk for heart disease . . . and high risk for breast cancer.

While there is no doubt that estrogen can do us a lot of good, the increased risk of breast cancer, small though it may be, is scary. Is that risk worth taking? There is no way to answer that question without scrutinizing your *personal* risks of osteoporosis, heart disease, and breast cancer.

Statistics tell us that our risk of dying from breast cancer is equal to the risk of dying from a hip fracture due to osteoporosis, while the risk of dying from a heart attack is MORE THAN TEN TIMES HIGHER than the threat presented by either breast cancer or osteoporosis. The odds of dying from uterine cancer as a result of taking estrogen replacement without protective progestin are lowest of all. But again it is important to remember that these odds are derived from population studies, not your personal health profile.

The questions we are faced with as menopause nears are perplexing. Do we have to choose between our bones and our breasts or can we protect both? Just how much does estrogen replacement increase the risk of breast cancer? Is there any way to minimize it? Does a family history of breast cancer mean you shouldn't take estrogen even if your risk of osteoporosis is high? How do you calculate your risk of breast cancer? And how does heart disease fit into the picture?

SPECIAL CIRCUMSTANCES

On a lesser scale there are questions that may tip the balance one way or another for many women. What if you have estrogen-fed fibroid tumors of the uterus? Will they grow if you take estrogen? Women with endometriosis face a similar dilemma, since estrogen can aggravate their condition.

Estrogen replacement is also an important consideration for any woman contemplating a hysterectomy and the removal of her ovaries. If you are premenopausal, the surgery will mean "instant" menopause and will have major implications for the future of your bones, your heart, and your sex life. Will estrogen replacement overcome all the potential problems? What happens if you have had a hysterectomy and your ovaries are left in place? If you don't have a uterus and don't get periods, how will you know when menopause arrives? If you feel you need estrogen, when should you begin to take it?

In making your decision you must also factor in quality of life considerations posed by the symptoms of menopause. Estrogen does a terrific job of banishing hot flashes, insomnia, and a host of other disturbing phenomena. What symptoms can you expect to develop at menopause? How bad will they be? What else besides estrogen is available to help you cope?

In the past, most women had only the experience of their friends ' and female relatives to draw on to judge whether what happened to them—or was about to happen—was normal. Today, results of a growing number of scientific studies are giving us welcome new insights into the duration and severity of the physical symptoms we may encounter.

DECIDING FOR YOURSELF

As you read the chapters ahead, you may be disturbed that so many questions about estrogen replacement remain unanswered. These gaps in information have led to charges that estrogen is being heavily promoted to women without solid evidence that it prevents heart disease and despite concerns that it may account in part for the rising rate of breast cancer. At the same time, enthusiasts minimize the risks and offer reassurances based more on wishful thinking than clear-cut scientific data. A more balanced view recognizes estrogen as an imperfect drug that can enhance women's health but also presents some risks.

One of the leading researchers in the field, Ronald Ross, M.D., of the University of Southern California, neatly summed up the dilemma we face: "Women have to be alert to the fact that there are risks and benefits. We know that the net effect of taking estrogen is reduced mortality (longer life spans), but that may not be true for the individual woman, especially the one who gets breast cancer. At this point, we just have to educate patients about the size of the equation and let them decide for themselves."

Sobering words. In the chapters ahead, I have tried to present the benefits and risks of estrogen replacement even-handedly. After all of my research, I have no "position" on estrogen replacement, no case to make pro or con. I do think that some doctors are recklessly encouraging women to take estrogen and that many women should avoid it at all costs and that others really need it and would be foolish not to take it.

Some of the risks you will be reading about are very disturbing and must be taken seriously, but, on a more positive note, none of us should lose sight of the benefits to be gained.

ⓉⓌⓄ

Menopause

MENOPAUSE PROBABLY IS not an event you have anticipated with enthusiasm. Like it or not, in our youth-centered culture, menopause represents decline. It is an undeniable marker of aging. Perhaps for that reason menopause is not a subject we dwell upon in advance. Some women look forward to an end to the inconvenience of menstruation, but most of us don't spend much time contemplating the other physical changes that will occur. In fact, a great many women have no clear idea of what to expect. As I spoke to women about menopause and its aftermath, I began to suspect that many harbored a secret belief that the changes it brings "can't happen to me." Nature's master plan for women doesn't seem any more welcome when menopause looms than it was nearly forty years earlier when, as little girls, we learned, with initial disbelief, that we could look forward to menstruating for most of our adult lives.

Menstruation was a major health event only insofar as it signaled the onset of our reproductive years. Menopause means far more than an end to fertility. It is a critical turning point in our well-being. Some of the effects of this shift in hormonal gears may become uncomfortably apparent as estrogen levels decline. The most devastating consequence—bone loss—probably will not be obvious for many years.

Nature constructed us as baby-making machines, and, in that respect, at menopause we become obsolete. The hormones that have governed our reproductive systems for almost forty years are signing off. Depleted of their inventory of eggs, our ovaries are going out of business. Most women have no desire to have babies after age fifty (although if you are determined to do so, it no longer is impossible), so the loss of fertility is not the emotional wrench doctors once believed it to be. The bad part has to do with the rest of our bodies. Unfortunately, the hormones responsible for the maintenance of the baby-making apparatus play a major role in our general health and well-being. In a sense, they gave us a free ride health wise for about fifty years.

ESTROGEN

You became a woman the instant an X chromosome from your mother met an X from your father at conception. (If your father had supplied a Y chromosome, you would have been a boy and, at this stage of your life, would probably be reading a book on how to lower your cholesterol.) By the fifth month of pregnancy the ovaries of a female fetus contain approximately 6 million eggs. By birth, this number has dropped to about 2 million. And by puberty the total is down to about 400,000. Every egg a woman produces has been with her since before her own birth.

During childhood, estrogen remains quiescent. But at about age seven or eight, hormones released by the pituitary prompt the ovaries to rev up estrogen production. In response to estrogen a young girl's breasts begin to bud and her secondary sexual characteristics begin to emerge (pubic and underarm hair begin to grow). The final event in this transformation is the arrival of menstruation, a signal that puberty is over.

Your mother probably told you that when you began to menstruate you had become capable of having a baby. That's not strictly true. Most girls don't begin to ovulate until a few years after menstruation begins.

The complex hormonal choreography controlling the menstrual cycle is set in motion by gonadotropin releasing hormone (GnRH), a hormone released by the hypothalamus, the control center in the brain. GnRH signals the pituitary to release follicle stimulating hormone (FSH). True to its name, FSH stimulates development of an estrogen-secreting follicle in the ovary. Every month a dozen or more follicles begin to mature, but, most of the time, only one completes the process. When estrogen production peaks, the pituitary responds by releasing luteinizing hormone (LH), which prompts ovulation, the point at which the egg bursts forth from the follicle and begins its journey through the fallopian tubes to the uterus. If the egg encounters a sperm en route and fertilization takes place, the resulting zygote, or fertilized egg, continues on to the uterus where it will implant itself, establishing a pregnancy. If conception does not occur, the egg breaks down and dissolves.

During the first half of the menstrual cycle, estrogen stimulates cells in the endometrium, the lining of the uterus, in preparation for pregnancy. This results in the thickening of the endometrium with a nourishing cushion of blood and tissue. At ovulation, another hormone comes into play. After the egg begins its journey, the ruptured follicle takes on a new role. It changes into the corpus luteum (Latin for "yellow body," the color the follicle assumes after ovulation). Then it begins to secrete progesterone, a hormone that regulates the action of estrogen. If pregnancy does not occur, progesterone production ceases and, in response, the endometrium sheds its buildup of blood and tissue as menstruation. As soon as this process is complete, the whole cycle starts all over again.

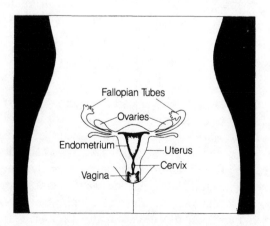

Source: What You Need to Know About Cancer of the Uterus, National Cancer Institute.

AN ALL-AROUND HORMONE

Estrogen gets a lot of the credit for the good health women enjoy before menopause. Although it is primarily a reproductive hormone, it seems to play important, if somewhat mysterious, roles elsewhere in the body. Estrogen facilitates absorption of calcium from the digestive system for use in bone building. It contributes to skin tone by helping maintain the collagen tissue that underlies skin. It may also be responsible for the fact that young women have a very low risk of heart disease. All we have to go on here is circumstantial evidence, the observation that heart disease is rare before menopause but increases afterward when estrogen levels decline. The risk of heart disease also rises among women whose ovaries have been removed in the course of a hysterectomy. This plus the fact that estrogen replacement reduces the risk of heart disease in women after menopause suggests, but does not prove, that estrogen is protective.

However, there is no doubt that estrogen is essential for the maintenance of healthy, functioning reproductive organs. As estrogen levels decline, the ovaries, uterus, and vagina begin to atrophy. The earliest and most obvious of these changes is vaginal dryness, which can make sexual intercourse uncomfortable, even painful. Some women say they are less interested in sex after menopause, but declining estrogen levels probably are not to blame here. Estrogen's role in sexual desire is not well understood. Other hormonal changes, perhaps a decrease in androgens, the male hormones believed to power the sex drive in both men and women, may be at fault.

THE CLIMACTERIC

Strictly speaking, menopause is a single event: your last menstrual period. But your body begins preparing for this change years before it occurs. Menopause does not mark the end of this transition. Instead, it is the midpoint in a process known as the climacteric, a gradual decline in estrogen production that begins in the late twenties or early thirties and ends fifteen or twenty years after menopause when estrogen levels finally bottom out. This change is so gradual and subtle that you probably did not notice any change in menstrual patterns until your midforties. Some women find their periods become shorter or sparser. For others, they get longer and heavier. Premenstrual symptoms may worsen . . . or disappear. Apart from menstrual changes, you are unlikely to experience any other physical signs of the climacteric. You probably do not ovulate as dependably as you did when you were younger, so if you postponed pregnancy until your late thirties or early forties, you are more likely to run into trouble conceiving than younger women. On the other hand, the fact that you may be ovulating erratically won't protect you from pregnancy. You cannot be positive that you won't get pregnant until two years after your last period!

THE MYSTERIES OF MENOPAUSE

Although we know what menopause is, no one knows for sure exactly what brings it about. Do estrogen levels have to fall below a certain threshold? Or do we have to run out of eggs? By the time we reach forty, the 400,000 follicles our ovaries contained at birth have decreased to less than 10,000. After that, the numbers decline rapidly. Sandra Richardson, M.D., a researcher at McGill University in Montreal, counted the follicles from ovaries removed during hysterectomies from seventeen healthy women aged forty-four to fifty-five. Those women who were having regular menstrual cycles at the time of surgery had about 1400 follicles. Women approaching menopause had about 142; postmenopausal women, none.

As ovulation becomes increasingly erratic during the climacteric, FSH levels begin to rise. In a young, fertile woman FSH is low, about 10 microinternational units (MIU) per milliliter of blood. As estrogen levels begin to decline, the pituitary increases the amount of FSH in an increasingly futile attempt to jump start failing ovaries, rev up estrogen production, and induce ovulation. When FSH levels pass 40 MIU per milliliter, you can consider yourself menopausal. Once they rise that high, they will never decline. FSH can be measured via a simple blood test that your doctor may perform to confirm that you have reached menopause.

TIMING

The average age of menopause in the United States is 51.4 years. But the *normal* age range is forty-five to fifty-five. If you want to know when you will reach menopause, ask your mother when she did. There is a pretty high hereditary correlation here. Perhaps our genes determine the number of eggs we're born with. If so, it would make sense that we would run out of eggs and estrogen at about the same time our mothers did.

Beyond this hereditary connection, researchers know very little about the timing of menopause, but a long-term study of Menstruation and Reproductive History at the University of Utah is beginning to yield some interesting information. Among the findings:

• Women who have short menstrual cycles (less than twenty-six days) reach menopause an average of 2.2 years earlier than those with cycles of thirty-three days or more.

• Women who had been pregnant reached menopause later than women who had never been pregnant.

• The more children you have, the later menopause occurs.

• Women who had five or more births reached menopause approximately one year later than women who never had given birth.

The study also verified earlier findings that showed that the age at which you started to menstruate has nothing to do with the age at which you stop.

PREMATURE MENOPAUSE

You can reach menopause ahead of schedule for a number of reasons. About 8 percent of all women stop menstruating before the age of forty. This so-called premature menopause appears to be under genetic control—it runs in the family, and you are more likely to stop menstruating early if your mother and other female relatives did, too.

You are also more likely to reach menopause five to ten years ahead of schedule if you are a smoker. No one has been able to explain why this occurs, although some researchers have speculated that smoking may speed up the aging process. Whatever the underlying reason, if you smoke, chances are you will reach menopause between five to ten years earlier than your mother (unless she, too, was a smoker) or other women in your family who do not smoke.

For unknown reasons, mothers of twins reach menopause about a year earlier than average.

In 18 to 30 percent of all cases, premature menopause (or, to use the medical term, premature ovarian failure) stems from an autoimmune disorder in which the body produces antibodies that alter normal ovarian function. Among these disorders are Graves' disease, Hashimoto's thyroiditis, Addison's disease, and myasthenia gravis.

Much more often, menopause arrives ahead of schedule when a woman's ovaries are removed in the course of a hysterectomy. This surgery is so common that about 25 percent of all women in the United States reach menopause on the operating table. Even when the ovaries are left in place, menopause tends to arrive early among women who have had hysterectomies. The only explanation here is an educated guess that the surgery itself affects the ovarian blood supply or disrupts some undiscovered hormonal pathway between the ovaries and uterus. (For a complete discussion of hysterectomy and its ramifications see Chapter Eight.)

Premature menopause represents a number of risks. The younger you are when estrogen levels decline to menopausal levels, the sooner you begin to lose bone mass and the more likely you are to suffer from osteoporosis later in life. And since heart disease in women seems to be related to declining estrogen levels, premature menopause may elevate your risk. Even more ominously, there is some preliminary medical evidence (which must be confirmed by further research) suggesting that early menopause often means early death. This news comes from a study of 5287 Seventh Day Adventists, a group that is about as close to ideal as you can get for research purposes because their diets are extremely healthy and, in general, they take very good care of themselves. The results, published in a 1990 issue of the *American Journal of Epidemiology*, showed that women who reached menopause naturally before the age of forty were twice as likely to die during the course of the study than women of the same age who reached menopause between the ages of fifty and fifty-four. The risk of early death was also higher than normal among those who reached menopause naturally between the ages of forty and forty-four and about 15 percent higher than normal among women who reached menopause between forty-five and forty-nine.

The researchers found that when menopause came early as a result of surgery—removal of the ovaries during a hysterectomy— there was *no* relationship between age of menopause and death. They also discovered that estrogen replacement did not increase longevity among women whose natural menopause occurred prematurely.

LATE MENOPAUSE

If early menopause is hazardous to health, late menopause should be just the opposite. Instead, it is a mixed blessing. The longer you continue to menstruate, the longer you enjoy the protective effects of estrogen on your bones and your heart. In that respect, late menopause is a valuable holding action—it postpones the inevitable changes. The longer your bones have the benefits of estrogen, the stronger they will be at a point in life when most women already have lost considerable bone mass. You will begin to lose bone, too, but when menopause is late, your bones will be stronger during your seventies and eighties than they would have been if you had reached menopause on time.

However, late menopause carries very serious risks: higher than normal rates of both breast and ovarian cancer. The danger appears to be related to the number of years of exposure to estrogen. The risk is particularly high among women who began to menstruate early and reached menopause late. Those who menstruate for more than forty years—say, from age eleven to age fifty-five—are at particularly high risk of both diseases.

There is a big exception to this general rule: women who took birth control pills or had multiple pregnancies seem to be at lower risk of ovarian cancer. Both the pill and pregnancy may give the ovaries a needed respite from monthly hormonal stimulation. No one knows why late menopause increases the risk of breast cancer, although here, too, the problem may be the length of exposure to estrogen. The birth control pill does not offer the same protection against breast cancer as it does against ovarian cancer.

PERIMENOPAUSE

Although most women don't notice any changes coinciding with the gradual drop in estrogen levels that accompanies the climacteric, perimenopause—the year or two leading up to menopause—is a different story. Now, changes in your menstrual pattern become obvious. Instead of arriving on schedule every month your periods may begin a few days early or a few days late. Eventually, they begin arriving a few weeks late. They may be shorter—or longer—

than usual. And the flow may be lighter—or heavier—than it once was. There are no rules governing perimenopause. You can skip your period for two or three (or six!) months only to have it go right back on schedule for another few months. It may start and stop then start again.

This menstrual chaos stems from fluctuating hormone levels brought about by ovaries that are less and less capable of generating estrogen. You probably are not ovulating, so you are not producing progesterone to round out the cycle and induce menstruation. Our bodies don't easily accept or adapt to these changes. The pituitary continues to dispatch LH and FSH, but this biochemical effort to restore ovarian hormone production is a losing battle.

During this period, the estrogen you still produce can stimulate the endometrium to thicken in preparation for pregnancy, but if you don't ovulate, there will be no progesterone and no timely period. Instead, your "period" arrives arbitrarily and can be alarmingly heavy. While this is not unusual among women approaching menopause, knowing that it falls within the realm of "normal" doesn't make it any easier to deal with. Your doctor may prescribe progesterone (or more precisely, a synthetic progesterone called progestin) to bring the bleeding under control and put you back on a manageable monthly menstrual schedule until you reach menopause (you will know when you get there because despite taking the progestin you won't get a period).

Some women who have had a lifetime of trouble-free periods develop premenstrual syndrome (PMS) in the years leading up to menopause. Conversely, women who have been plagued by PMS through the years may find their symptoms lessening or disappearing as menopause approaches. Since PMS itself is something of a medical mystery, there is no good explanation for why it gets worse or better as menopause approaches. Fluctuating hormone levels would seem to be the obvious explanation, but researchers who have studied PMS have found no hormonal differences between affected women (even those with severe, disabling symptoms) and those who have no difficulties at all.

Perimenopause usually lasts about one year, but it can go on for much longer. Some women just stop menstruating without going through any irregularities at all, but most of us will have to deal with a year or more of uncertainty.

MENOPAUSE

You won't know for sure that you have reached menopause until one year after your last period. Chances are that once you pass the six-month mark you won't menstruate again, but you can't be sure of that. You also can't be sure that you are not ovulating, and if you do, you can get pregnant. This happens often enough for doctors to warn against abandoning contraception for a year after the last period . . . unless, of course, you wouldn't object to a little surprise.

Once it is a fait accompli, menopause can bring about changes in the way we feel and look. Some can be chalked up to the aging process, not menopause per se. But life without estrogen is going to be different.

SEX AFTER MENOPAUSE

When menopause was a taboo topic, nobody talked about the effect it had on a woman's sex life. Or if the subject did come up it was shrouded in optimism. The consensus seemed to be that sex improved after menopause because women no longer had to worry about pregnancy. But no one mentioned vaginal dryness, the fact that women don't lubricate as readily when estrogen levels are low. No one warned us that, in time, without estrogen, vaginal walls become paper thin. The question of sexual desire after menopause is also somewhat confusing. Does our sex drive begin to wane as some studies seem to indicate? Or is something else going on? Does the fact that sex becomes increasingly less comfortable explain the lessening of interest? Or does diminished desire have something to do with the men—or lack of them—in our lives?

Not every woman suffers from vaginal dryness after menopause—at least not immediately. Here, we seem to be dealing to some degree with a "use it or lose it" situation. Women who maintain active sex lives seem to have less of a problem (or no problem at all) in this area, while women whose sex lives are sporadic or nonexistent can run into trouble even before menopause arrives. But, as with anything concerning menopause, vaginal dryness as a response to declining estrogen levels is highly individualized. If it becomes a problem, it can be more than a minor nuisance.

The impact of this change was made clear to me in chillingly succinct terms by a woman who had a terrible time with menopausal symptoms: "The vaginal dryness was unbelievable. Sex was torture. It was like being rubbed by an emery board." We are not talking here about a repressed spinster with a bad attitude or a weary wife with a miserable marriage. The woman who told me this is unmarried but involved in a long-term relationship. She is sophisticated, attractive, athletic, unwilling to sacrifice her sex life. Her solution was estrogen replacement.

Estrogen replacement usually can overcome the dryness problem (although one woman told me she needs a vaginal lubricant in addition to estrogen). However, there is no good evidence to show that estrogen replacement will invigorate a flagging sex drive. The researcher who has done the most work in this area, Barbara Sherwin, Ph.D., of McGill University in Montreal, maintains that "estrogen definitely does not affect sexuality." She has been championing the use of androgen, a male hormone, to enhance the libido of postmenopausal women.

In 1985 Dr. Sherwin and her team of researchers in Canada found that a combination of estrogen and androgen did wonders to restore libido among women whose ovaries had been removed in the course of hysterectomies. Their studies showed that the combination of the two hormones enhanced the women's sexual desire, arousal, and fantasy. Further studies have confirmed these findings and have compared the effect on sexuality of estrogen replacement alone to estrogen replacement plus androgen.

For one of her studies, Dr. Sherwin recruited women who had been taking estrogen and complained about lack of sexual desire. Adding the androgen to the estrogen eliminated the problem for 80 percent of the women participating.

So far, the only androgen side effect noted has been the growth of hair on the upper lip or chin, a problem Dr. Sherwin says can be solved by adjusting the dose. In addition to its effect on sexuality, Dr. Sherwin has shown that adding androgen to estrogen replacement "consistently induces a greater sense of well-being and higher energy level and alleviates feelings of tiredness and lethargy often experienced by postmenopausal women." Androgen is available in tablet form, and combined with estrogen in a single tablet. However, it is not widely prescribed, perhaps because women don't know about it or do not discuss postmenopausal changes in sexual desire with their doctors.

For some women, lack of interest in sex may have to do with

the lack of a partner. In their book *Sexual Desire Disorders* psychotherapists Sandra R. Leiblum, Ph.D., and Raymond C. Rosen, Ph.D., suggest that, unlike men, women can put their sex drives on "hold" indefinitely if no attractive man is available. They also cite studies showing that lesbian couples engage in sex far less frequently than heterosexual couples (once a month or less), which, they say, may indicate that the female sex drive idles in low gear absent an available male partner.

THE UTERUS AND OVARIES

After menopause, the uterus and ovaries begin to shrink. You probably won't notice any symptoms as a result of these changes, although uterine contractions that some women experience at orgasm may not be as powerful or pleasurable as they once were. Although the ovaries get smaller, they continue to secrete some estrogen plus a hormone, called androstenedione, which is converted into estrogen by fat cells.

After menopause, the incidence of both uterine (endometrial) and ovarian cancer begins to increase. Of the two, ovarian cancer is a much greater threat because it cannot be detected until it is advanced. The only symptom of this disease may be an enlargement in a postmenopausal ovary. For this reason, it is vital to continue with regular gynecological check-ups after menopause whether or not you choose to take estrogen replacement. Every year, about 21,000 American women develop ovarian cancer.

Uterine cancer is much less of a problem because it does cause early symptoms—unexpected bleeding. Because it can be detected early, it usually can be cured. One woman in every thousand will develop uterine cancer this year. Risks are higher among those who take estrogen replacement unless they also take progestin to counteract estrogen's effects on the endometrium.

URINARY PROBLEMS

Declining estrogen levels affect the urinary tract and bladder as well as the vagina. Deprived of estrogen the epithelial cells lining the urinary tract begin to degenerate. As a result, the muscles responsible for bladder control weaken. This can lead to stress incontinence, a loss of urine when you cough, sneeze, or laugh. Estrogen replacement can restore the urinary tract lining to its former strength and solve the incontinence problem. An alternative solution is muscle strengthening via an exercise program developed in the 1950s by A. M. Kegel, M.D. These exercises are described in Chapter Eight.

Postmenopausal changes in the urinary tract also predispose some women to recurrent bladder infections. Estrogen replacement helps with this problem, too, but there are other steps you can take. The more often you urinate, the less likely you are to develop infections—the bugs that cause them thrive in concentrated urine. You will urinate more frequently if you drink a lot of water (eight glasses per day is ideal). The water also dilutes the urine, making it less receptive to infection-causing bacteria. Cranberry juice can help, too, because it acidifies the chemistry of the urinary tract making it less hospitable to bacteria.

SKIN CHANGES

Estrogen deprivation is supposed to be bad for your skin, but extravagant claims and general impressions to the contrary, there is no proof that estrogen replacement will stave off the effects of aging. In fact, the package inserts that come with postmenopausal estrogens clearly state that there is no evidence that estrogen will keep skin soft and supple or keep you feeling young.

It is true that naturally produced estrogen does play a role in skin maintenance. When you are young and your ovaries are producing plenty of estrogen, skin is firm, moist, and well padded with a layer of fat that gives skin its youthful contour. But your genes and the amount of time you have spent in the sun have much more to do with the way your skin ages than the amount of estrogen circulating in your blood. Don't expect estrogen replacement to undo sun damage, which is much more devastating to skin than estrogen deprivation. The plentiful supply of natural estrogen you have before menopause can't prevent the damage to collagen, the skin's supporting fibers, inflicted by years of sun exposure. If you have any doubts on this score, compare the skin on your hands to the skin on the inside of your upper arm (an area that doesn't get a lot of sun). The difference probably will shock you, and it will certainly show you what is primarily responsible for the way your skin looks today.

The general impression that women on estrogen replacement have better skin than women who take no hormones has not been investigated scientifically. But there may be another explanation for the difference. Since women who take estrogen are usually better educated, thinner, healthier, and more affluent than women who don't take estrogen, they may also take pretty good care of their skin.

This skin question is kind of subjective anyway. Good skin may be all in the eye of the beholder. I know plenty of women with great skin who don't take hormones and plenty with not-so-good skin who do take them. I personally am counting on heredity and sunscreens to protect me in the skin department. Believe me, if your skin needs help, Retin A will do you more good than estrogen replacement.

HAIR

After menopause you may find hair sprouting where you don't want it—on your face. This unwelcome change has to do with the balance of hormones and the fact that the male hormones produced in your body become more influential once estrogen levels fall. Estrogen replacement can help here, but, of course, there are other ways of solving this problem. Electrolysis will get rid of the hair permanently. Waxing or tweezing may be all you need.

You may also notice that underarm and pubic hair becomes more sparse after menopause. This change is definitely related to estrogen—after all, these secondary sexual characteristics developed during puberty when estrogen was transforming you from a girl into a woman.

The hair on your head may become thinner, coarser, and drier, a change that estrogen replacement will not affect. Not to worry: look around. There are plenty of attractive older women whose hair looks terrific.

WEIGHT

Most women do gain weight after menopause, and it is harder to lose unwanted pounds. You may also notice that your weight is distributed differently, less in your hips and breasts and more in your upper back and abdomen. There is no hormonal magic that will change this picture. Even estrogen replacement's greatest boosters make no claims here. If you want to be slim, there's only one way to do it: eat less and exercise more.

A LITTLE OPTIMISM, PLEASE

All these changes sound pretty dismal and they do suggest that we may have to work harder to feel good and look good. At the same time, it is important to remember that all the changes menopause brings don't develop overnight. I decided time is still on our side the day I found a picture of my mother and two of my aunts. They looked great. Vibrant, healthy, happy, pretty. From the date on the picture I figured out how old they were at the time: fifty-seven, fifty-eight, and fifty-nine.

🅣🅗🅡🅔🅔

Estrogen

ESTROGEN REPLACEMENT is not a new idea. Premarin, the most widely prescribed estrogen for menopausal symptoms, has been on the market since 1942. In its press materials, Wyeth Ayerst, the manufacturer, boasts that Premarin is "the most widely studied and prescribed estrogen product in the world" and that approximately 6 million American women take it. Premarin and Estraderm, a Band-Aid-like patch that delivers estrogen through the skin, are the two major competitors in the menopause market today. And, make no mistake, this is a huge market that is getting bigger every day: during the next decade the number of women reaching the menopausal years between forty-five and fifty-four will total 19 million. Add that to the 43 million women already past menopause and you begin to see why "the change," its symptoms, long-term effects, and the estrogen question have suddenly emerged from secrecy to become the hottest topic in women's health.

WHAT ESTROGEN CAN DO

For the record, estrogen is approved by the U.S. Food and Drug Administration (FDA) for treatment of three conditions:

- Hot flashes and night sweats, known in medical parlance as "vasomotor symptoms." (Vasomotor refers to the fact that blood vessels near the skin dilate in response to the temperature change.)
- Vaginal dryness (you may see this referred to in medicalese as "atrophic vaginitis").
- The prevention and treatment of osteoporosis.

Despite evidence that estrogen replacement can protect women against heart disease, it is not approved by the FDA for this purpose. And, contrary to what many women (and some doctors) believe, there is no evidence that estrogen replacement protects the skin from the effects of aging. Similarly, there is no scientific proof that estrogen prevents or relieves menopausal depression if, indeed, depression at this stage of life differs at all from any other kind of depression (recent studies suggest that it does not). The bottom line here is that although estrogen replacement will prevent or reverse symptoms brought on by declining levels of natural estrogen, it will not stop or even slow the clock on the aging process. The lingering impression (or desperate hope?) that estrogen replacement will keep women looking and feeling young may stem from negative attitudes toward menopause fostered by some doctors (one, a distinguished researcher who shall remain nameless, told me that women *smell* different after menopause). And if those doctors are as old as women reaching menopause in the early 1990s, they came of age, professionally, in the swinging sixties when estrogen was widely viewed and heavily promoted as a "youth pill."

"FEMININE FOREVER"

The women's health sensation of 1966 was the book *Feminine Forever* by Robert Wilson, M.D., a Brooklyn physician with strong financial ties to drug companies that made and marketed postmenopausal estrogens. Wilson painted a vividly dismal picture of menopause (he termed it "living decay") and listed symptoms ranging from hot flashes and night sweats to crying spells, dizziness, chronic indigestion, backache, and even neuroses and suicidal thoughts. At the same time, drug companies were aggressively promoting estrogen to doctors often via medical magazine advertisements showing dowdy women looking just this side of sanity pictured with husbands who clearly were nonplussed by the changes in their wives presumably induced by menopause. Estrogen, the ad copy suggested, would set these haggard women to rights. The upshot of this hype was that millions of women began to take estrogen, some of them years before menopause.

At the time, hot flashes were widely regarded as a psychosomatic symptom, a reflection of the mental and emotional turmoil menopause was believed to inflict. Happily, we have passed beyond all that. We know that hot flashes are physiological, not psychological, and that as a rule, women don't fall apart mentally, physically, and emotionally at menopause. But the "youth pill" mystique still surrounds estrogen. With no evidence to back them up doctors often suggest to women that without estrogen we will lose our vitality, our looks, our sexuality.

ESTROGEN AND THE ENDOMETRIUM

As early as 1947, almost twenty years before *Feminine Forever*, the first reports began to appear in medical literature that estrogen's effects on the endometrium, the lining of the uterus, could be dangerous. In premenopausal women estrogen stimulates the endometrium in the first half of the menstrual cycle, thickening it in preparation for pregnancy. As you will remember, in the second half of the cycle both estrogen and progesterone are present. If pregnancy does not take place, progesterone levels drop and the endometrial buildup is shed as menstruation.

But what happens to the endometrium if it is stimulated by estrogen year in and year out after menopause when there is no natural progesterone around to complete the cycle? In time, this constant stimulation can lead to a condition known as hyperplasia, an overgrowth and proliferation of endometrial cells that can lead to cancer. The only symptom of an overstimulated endometrium is bleeding, and, in fact, it was the high rate of bleeding among women taking estrogen that began to suggest as long ago as the 1940s that estrogen was causing trouble.

Finally, in 1975, a study published in the *New England Journal of Medicine* showed that women who took estrogen replacement had five to fourteen times the normal rate of endometrial cancer. This news had an immediate and predictable impact on women who were taking estrogen: most of them stopped. (The cancer scare did not affect women who had had hysterectomies: you can't get endometrial cancer when you don't have a uterus.) The cancer risk was highest among women who had taken high doses of estrogen for five years or more.

ENDOMETRIAL CANCER

Endometrial cancer is the most common gynecological cancer. The American Cancer Society estimates that it develops in one of every one thousand women each year for an annual total of about 32,000 cases. That translates to a lifetime risk of two cases per hundred (in the course of a lifetime, two out of every hundred women will get endometrial cancer as opposed to one out of every seventy women who will get ovarian cancer, the second most common gynecological malignancy). The incidence of breast cancer is much higher, about 180,000 cases per year, which works out to a lifetime risk of one woman in nine. Normally, risks of endometrial cancer are highest among women who are 30 percent or more overweight. While obesity is by far the strongest risk factor, there are others:

• A history of infertility.
• A history of failure to ovulate or menstruate regularly.
• A history of polycystic ovarian disease (a condition resulting from a hormonal irregularity that leads to development of many abnormal ovarian cysts).
• Endometrial hyperplasia, an abnormal thickening of the uterine lining.
• A history of breast, ovarian, or colon cancer.
• A family history of endometrial cancer (specifically, an affected mother or daughter).
• High blood pressure.

Endometrial cancer is most common among women between the ages of fifty and seventy. The average age at diagnosis is sixty.

Interestingly, women who have taken birth control pills seem to have a reduced risk of endometrial cancer.

Before endometrial cancer develops, a progression of three distinct changes must take place in the endometrium. These changes, all benign, are various stages of *hyperplasia*, an abnormal proliferation of endometrial cells that can cause unexpected uterine bleeding. The first stage, *cystic hyperplasia*, rarely leads to cancer. The second, *adenomatous hyperplasia*, and the third, *atypical hyperplasia*, are more worrisome, but all three can usually be treated successfully with progestin.

Endometrial cancer typically causes vaginal bleeding, a symptom signaling trouble, even when the disease is in its earliest stages. If detected in the first of its four stages, when cancer is localized, chances for a cure are excellent: about 93 percent of all women survive for more than five years. Advanced endometrial cancer, which has spread beyond the uterus to other parts of the body, is more difficult to treat and cure. Here, the five-year survival rate is about 27 percent. Despite the increased number of endometrial cancer cases seen during the 1960s and 1970s, the death rate from this disease has declined by 69 percent since the late 1950s. Perhaps, as some studies have suggested, endometrial cancer among women who have been taking estrogen replacement is less aggressive than it is when it occurs among women who have not been on estrogen.

Diagnosis

In addition to abnormal bleeding (which includes spotting), a watery discharge with an odor may also indicate endometrial cancer and may occur before any bleeding develops. Diagnosis usually requires a biopsy in which samplings of endometrial cells are scraped out for laboratory testing. By all reports an endometrial biopsy is no fun, but it isn't surgery either. A properly performed endometrial biopsy, which can be done in a doctor's office, is as accurate as the other diagnostic method, a D & C (dilatation and curettage), a minor surgical procedure performed in the hospital under general anesthesia. During a D & C, the cervix is dilated and the uterine lining scraped with an instrument called a curette. The tissue is then examined to determine if the source of the problem is hyperplasia, endometrial cancer, or something else. (Bleeding can be due to endometrial polyps or benign fibroid tumors of the uterus.) If the results indicate hyperplasia, treatment with progestin usually takes care of the problem. When a malignancy is found, treatment will require a hysterectomy and removal of the cervix, ovaries, and fallopian tubes. Sometimes, radiation therapy is given before or after surgery. Women who have had endometrial cancer cannot take estrogen replacement afterward because of the possibility that the estrogen might prompt the growth of any remaining cancer cells. However, in some cases where doctors are confident that no cancer

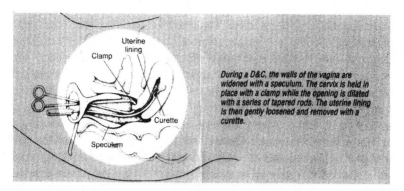

During a D&C, the walls of the vagina are widened with a speculum. The cervix is held in place with a clamp while the opening is dilated with a series of tapered rods. The uterine lining is then gently loosened and removed with a curette.

Source: Cancer of the Uterus, American College of Obstetricians and Gynecologists, 1992.

remains, women may be able to take estrogen to relieve severe menopausal symptoms or to protect against osteoporosis.

PROGESTIN: PROS AND CONS

The solution to the endometrial cancer crisis for women taking estrogen replacement has been the addition of progestin. Not only can this hormone eliminate hyperplasia, it can prevent it from developing by counteracting the effects of estrogen on the uterine lining. The theory here is simple: taking progestin will stimulate the menstrual cycle. You take estrogen for twelve days then add progestin for twelve to fourteen more days, then quit taking both drugs. When the progestin is withdrawn, the endometrium reacts the way it did before menopause: it sheds the estrogen-stimulated buildup. The addition of progestin appears to eliminate the increased risk of endometrial cancer posed by estrogen replacement. In fact, some studies have shown that women taking both hormones have a lower than normal risk of endometrial cancer. However, in general, adding progestin eliminates only the *additional* risk that estrogen poses. Women taking both estrogen and progestin have developed endometrial cancer, but this is rare, and, for the most part, experts say, the affected women were at very high risk because they were obese.

Although taking progestin does appear to solve the endometrial cancer problem, its use raises some troubling questions. When progestin was added to estrogen replacement, there had been no long-term studies to determine whether it posed any health risks. The studies that *were* done showed that it did not counteract estrogen's effects on hot flashes or interfere with the protection against osteoporosis. The only negative finding seemed to be the resumption of monthly bleeding, a very unpopular development. But bleeding is a minor inconvenience compared with more recent indications that progestin may increase the risk of breast cancer and partly counteract the protection estrogen appears to provide against heart disease. Some researchers now worry that progestin is doing women more harm than good. Stay tuned on this subject. There should be some very interesting developments in the near future.

BREAST CANCER

Questions about the impact of estrogen replacement on breast cancer risk are so important and, for many women, so decisive that I am devoting a whole chapter to it (see Chapter Seven). At this writing, it appears that estrogen replacement does increase the risk of breast cancer slightly, particularly among women who have been treated for ten years or more, and this increased risk may be magnified by taking progestin.

WHO CANNOT TAKE ESTROGEN

You definitely cannot take estrogen if you have any of the following conditions:
  • Breast cancer.
  • Endometrial cancer.
  • Seriously impaired liver function.
  • A history of phlebitis (an inflammation of a vein involving a blood clot) or a disorder involving an embolism (blood clot), particularly if it was related to taking birth control pills.
  • Abnormal or unexplained vaginal bleeding.
  As I explained previously, if you have a history of endometrial cancer—you had it more than three years ago and it has not recurred—some doctors might prescribe estrogen for severe menopausal symptoms. Since endometrial cancer usually can be cured when caught early, taking estrogen after successful treatment when

you are fairly certain you are cancer free may not be a big risk. Whether women who have had breast cancer should ever take estrogen is a much trickier question. Breast cancer is often very slow growing, so recurrences may not show up until fifteen years or more after it first developed. However, some doctors do prescribe estrogen in vaginal cream to women who have had breast cancer in order to relieve vaginal dryness.

Although we tend to focus on cancer, estrogen replacement presents some other risks, which, while not life-threatening, can be troublesome if they occur.

GALLSTONES

Doctors describe the typical gallbladder patient as "female, fair, fat, and forty." Making it to menopause without gallbladder problems doesn't mean you are home free, and estrogen replacement appears to more than double the risk of gallstones.

Gallstones are made up of cholesterol and other fatty substances in bile. They usually cause no problem and produce no symptoms. As a result, you don't know you have them and don't have to do anything about them. The only time gallstones cause trouble is when they try to move out of the gallbladder and get stuck in the duct through which bile (wastes from the liver) flows from the gallbladder to the intestines. A trapped gallstone produces intense pain in the upper right side of the abdomen or, sometimes, between the shoulder blades. This pain, called biliary colic, will go away if the stone gets unstuck and either drops back into the gallbladder or gets pushed into the intestines. If pain persists and tests show you have gallstones, you probably will need surgery. (Luckily, gallbladder surgery today is not the big deal it used to be. Stones generally can be removed via a procedure called laparascopic cholecystectomy in which a long, thin instrument with a tiny viewing scope is inserted into the abdomen through a small incision. Other surgical instruments are inserted through other little incisions. Because of the small size of the incisions, the time spent in the hospital and convalescence are much shorter than they used to be when gallbladder surgery required opening the abdomen.) Some doctors believe that the increased risk of gallstones among women on estrogen replacement occurs only when the hormone is taken in pill form and must pass through the liver to enter the bloodstream. The estrogen patch was designed to overcome this problem and, in theory, should reduce the gallstone risk. However, so far, no studies have confirmed that it does.

FIBROIDS

Fibroid tumors of the uterus are benign growths affecting about 40 percent of all women. No one knows what causes fibroids, but they do seem to develop and grow only in the presence of estrogen. Most fibroids cause no symptoms and require no treatment. They are usually discovered during a routine pelvic exam, and as long as they don't get very large, cause bleeding or pain, or exert pressure on the bladder, they can safely be ignored.

The decline in estrogen production at menopause usually causes fibroids to shrink. But what happens to fibroids if you take estrogen replacement after menopause? They *usually* do not grow, but they could. If so, they probably will shrink if you go off estrogen. You won't be able to go back on so you will have to find alternative ways to deal with menopausal symptoms and the risks of osteoporosis and heart disease.

If fibroids get large enough to cause discomfort or block access to your ovaries during a pelvic exam, your doctor will probably recommend a hysterectomy. A number of less drastic alternatives are now available but may not be suitable for women past menopause. Large fibroids can be removed via myomectomy, an operation in which the fibroids are excised and the uterus left intact. (Myoma is medicalese for fibroid, hence "myomectomy," or removal of fibroids.) Fibroids often recur in young women, but usually don't return among those past forty.

Like hysterectomy, myomectomy is major surgery, requiring a week in the hospital and another six weeks convalescing at home. It is considered a more serious operation than a hysterectomy. Although there is no medical reason why a woman past menopause cannot have a myomectomy, it won't be easy to find a surgeon willing to perform the operation. Most doctors will insist that hysterectomy is more appropriate for women past childbearing age.

ENDOMETRIOSIS

The question of whether a woman who has endometriosis should take estrogen replacement is a particularly tricky one. This condition occurs when fragments of endometrial tissue migrate outside the uterus and implant elsewhere in the pelvic cavity. Despite the fact that it no longer is located in the uterus, the displaced tissue continues to behave like the endometrium, responding to estrogen and progesterone and bleeding every month right on schedule. The pain caused by this abnormal state of affairs can be disabling. Menopause is supposed to put an end to the worst of the symptoms. But what if women with endometriosis feel they need estrogen to protect against osteoporosis or combat vaginal dryness? Will the estrogen stimulate their displaced endometrial tissue and bring back the pain? What about the cancer risk? What is the effect of estrogen replacement on endometrial tissue that no longer is in the uterus?

Premenopausal women with endometriosis who have had their ovaries removed in the course of hysterectomy are not usually given estrogen replacement immediately after surgery as are most other premenopausal women. Some doctors advocate waiting three months, others say nine months, in hopes that any endometrial tissue left behind will atrophy and cease to respond to estrogen stimulation. Theoretically, a woman who has endometriosis and still has her uterus and ovaries could wait three to nine months before beginning estrogen replacement in hopes that there will be no return of symptoms. If you have endometriosis, this is a question that requires a lot of thought and discussion with your physician.

Another worry for women who have endometriosis is the question of whether estrogen replacement might lead to cancer in endometrial implants outside the uterus. Although this is extremely unlikely, it has happened. Like all the other estrogen questions, there are no easy answers here and no consensus among doctors about the correct course of action. If you have endometriosis and feel you need estrogen after menopause, your only option may be to wait a few months and then proceed with caution.

MIGRAINES

Migraine headaches are often associated with hormonal fluctuations that govern the menstrual cycle. Headaches may occur just before menstruation, about midway through the period, or at ovulation. These so-called hormonal headaches seem to stem from a drop in estrogen levels. However, they sometimes disappear during pregnancy when estrogen levels are continuously high. The effect of menopause is equally ambiguous: sometimes the headaches vanish, sometimes they get worse. Estrogen appears to affect the action of serotonin, a brain chemical that in turn affects production of endorphins, naturally produced pain killers. In addition to estrogen, yet another class of hormones, prostaglandins, seem to be involved in the migraines. Prostaglandins sensitize the nervous system to pain, light, and noise, thus accentuating headache symptoms. Estrogen replacement at menopause may worsen migraines, but adjustments in dosage can sometimes solve the problem. Although a history of migraines does not mean you cannot take estrogen, you may find that your headaches worsen and you cannot tolerate it.

HIGH BLOOD PRESSURE

Unlike the birth control pill, estrogen replacement does not appear to cause high blood pressure, but a conscientious doctor will take your pressure during every checkup. If your pressure does rise, your liver could be producing too much angiotensin, an enzyme sometimes associated with hypertension. If so, switching from oral estrogen to the patch could solve the problem.

🄵🄾🅄🅁

Hot Flashes
and Other Menopausal
Miseries

HOT FLASHES ARE THE MOST notorious and common symptom of menopause. Insomnia ranks second, and beyond that some of us experience a number of other changes in our feelings of well-being: depression, moodiness, memory lapses, joint pain, and a rare but bizarre skin tingling that, I'm told, feels like crawling insects.

Estrogen can relieve most but not all of these symptoms. The alternatives to estrogen are unreliable and unproven. The big surprise for me in this area was how few women felt they needed any help at all. I found no one who was depressed, no one who complained of memory problems or joint pains. The more women I talked to the more I began to suspect that for most of us menopausal symptoms will definitely be tolerable. But, as I've said before, my survey was far from scientific, and, as you will see, an unlucky minority of menopausal women do have a terrible time.

HOT FLASHES

Fredi Kronenberg, a researcher at Columbia University's College of Physicians and Surgeons, is the only scientist in the United States spending full time studying hot flashes. She knows much more about them than most physicians. Dr. Kronenberg can tell you that no rules apply to these common symptoms of menopause, at least no rules that researchers have discovered. When it comes to hot flashes, every woman is a law unto herself. You may reach menopause at the same time as your mother but don't bother to ask her about hot flashes: heredity does not seem to operate here. There is no way to predict whether you will have hot flashes, how often you will have them, how severe they will be, or how long they will last. Estrogen replacement usually will relieve them, but no one knows why. Other perplexing questions about estrogen and hot flashes have yet to be answered satisfactorily: does estrogen mask hot flashes or suppress them? Will the flashes return if you quit taking estrogen? If they do, will they be more or less troublesome?

Not so very long ago, doctors told complaining women that hot flashes were "all in your head," the same popular line once used when the problem was menstrual cramps. We know enough about hot flashes today to be sure that they are physiological, probably a response to declining estrogen levels, but researchers still have many more questions than answers about them. In a 1990 review of current research on the subject, Dr. Kronenberg listed what remains to be learned:

. . . *the average age at which hot flashes begin, factors that influence the age at hot flash onset and specific triggers of hot flashes. We do not know why hot flashes last only a few months in some women, while in others they persist for years or never occur at all. . . . We still do not understand fully the physiology of hot flashes, the mechanism by which a decline in estrogen levels leads to hot flashes or precisely how estrogen or any other therapy works to relieve them.*

An Unmistakable Sensation

If you have ever had a hot flash, you have no doubt about what it is. It is an unmistakable sensation that may come as a big surprise, but, trust me, you will know what it is when it happens. In an interview for an article published in *Allure* magazine in January 1992, Jane Fonda described her first hot flash: She and Ted Turner were in Athens attending a sound and light show at the Acropolis. "I started feeling this kind of burning tingling all down my fingers and chest, and I thought, 'I'm having a goddam hot flash. I can't believe it.' I was absolutely enthralled. I mean, I thought it was hysterical it was happening there."

"Enthralled" is probably not the term most women would use to describe their reactions to the first hot flash, although many remember the occasion as clearly as Fonda. "I was a guest lecturer teaching a class at my alma mater," said Sandy, a public relations executive and mother of two daughters, "suddenly I began to feel hot. I was sweating like crazy. I took off my jacket and then my scarf. I was beginning to wonder how much further I could go when I began to cool off."

Hot flashes typically begin with a momentary premonition or aura that signals their approach. This sensation may be a change in heart rate, a feeling of heat, or a flutter of anxiety. When Fredi Kronenberg asked women about this aura as part of a survey on hot flashes, 32 percent of her 438 respondents said they "just know" when a hot flash is impending. This "aura" or premonition is sometimes referred to as the "flash" and the heat wave that follows as the "flush." In general, however, the British use the term "hot flushes" while most Americans speak of "flashes."

The flash itself usually is described as a sensation of heat that begins in the chest and back and moves up (but not down) the body to the neck and head. Scientific studies of what happens physiologically during hot flashes show that the heart beats faster, blood vessels dilate, and skin temperature rises. Flashes typically are accompanied by some sweating, flushing, or anxiety and may be followed by chills. The women participating in Fredi Kronenberg's study also reported that during their hot flashes they felt irritated, annoyed, frustrated. Some mentioned a sense of panic or feelings of suffocation. A few even said they felt suicidal.

Most women sweat during hot flashes, but this can range from a barely detectable film of moisture on the forehead and neck to profuse perspiration that requires changing clothes and, if flashes occur at night, bed linen. The timing of hot flashes also contributes to some confusion on the subject. "Night sweats" are often included on some lists of menopausal symptoms, but the only real distinction between hot flashes and night sweats seems to be whether or not you are in bed and the lights are out when the heat goes on.

No Apparent Pattern

Despite the years she has devoted to the study of hot flashes, Fredi Kronenberg has not been able to discern a pattern to them. The results of her study will give you an idea of the difficulty here. The women participating ranged in age from twenty-nine to eighty-two, although the mean age was 49.5 for women who reached menopause naturally and 43.7 for those who had had their ovaries removed. Contrary to what we always have been told about hot flashes, half of the women in Dr. Kronenberg's study began having them while their menstrual cycles were still regular or just becoming irregular. The rest reported that their flashes began within a year of menopause although a few said they had no flashes until two years later.

Dr. Kronenberg's study also showed that there was no time of day when the flashes are more or less frequent (although one long-suffering woman has been plagued with hot flashes every hour of every day since she had her ovaries removed in 1980!). Of the women participating who were having hot flashes during the course of the study, 87 percent had one or more per day. About one third reported more than ten per day but the range was enormous: anywhere from five to fifty. When asked to rate their flashes as "mild," "moderate," or "severe," 26 percent chose "severe" while one third of the group said their flashes were "variable in intensity."

Flashes were much more likely to be described as "severe" by three groups of women: (1) those whose ovaries had been removed; (2) those who had hysterectomies but retained their ovaries; and (3) those who were premenopausal. Perimenopausal women tended to rate their flashes as varied or of moderate intensity.

When asked to describe their flashes, 88.8 percent of all the women participating mentioned heat and 86.5 percent said they also perspired. Here's a list of other feelings the women reported:

Burning	37.9%
Flushing	79.5%
Pressure in head	27.6%
Pressure in chest	16.0%
Change in heart rate	40.4%
Anxiety	29.0%
Ill/nauseous	57.8%
Chills/clamminess	19.0%
Embarrassment	41.6%
Depression	37.7%
Suicidal	6.4%

Typically, hot flashes become less frequent and less intense over time. But there is no way to predict what "over time" really means.

One study cited by Dr. Kronenberg showed that 64 percent of the women participating had hot flashes for between one and five years; 26 percent for six to ten years, and 10 percent for more than eleven years. Hot flashes tend to be longer lasting among women who have had their ovaries removed.

Missing Links

When Dr. Kronenberg looked into what, other than menopause itself, predisposes women to hot flashes, she came up empty-handed. She found no association between hot flashes and employment status, social class, age, marital status, domestic workload, or the number of children a woman has had. The age at which you began to menstruate or the age at which you stop has nothing to do with whether or not you'll have hot flashes, how bad they will be, or how long they will last.

The *only* factor that seems to play any role at all is weight. The thinner you are, the more likely you are to have hot flashes. No one knows for sure why overweight women have less of a problem. But the explanation may be as simple as the fact that estrogen is produced in fat cells.

Curiously, culture appears to influence how women experience menopause. Japanese women suffer from hot flashes less often than women in Western societies. The same seems to be true of Indonesian women. Mayan women living in the Yucatan report no symptoms of menopause other than irregular periods. Fredi Kronenberg wonders whether women in these cultures really do not have hot flashes or if the flashes occur "but are either perceived differently or not attributed to menopause." There is also some speculation that hot flashes do not occur in societies where the diet is high in foods containing plant estrogens, but no studies have confirmed this.

THE ESTROGEN CONNECTION

The notion that an estrogen deficit causes hot flashes comes from observations that they usually occur when estrogen levels are low—after the ovaries are removed and as women approach menopause—and that they disappear when estrogen is replaced. Dr. Kronenberg wants to know why, if low estrogen is to blame, all menopausal women don't have hot flashes or why some women have hot flashes during pregnancy when estrogen levels are exceptionally high. So far, no other hormone or interplay of hormones has been linked to hot flashes.

Since estrogen does play a role in regulating the body's internal thermometer as well as the nervous system and the vascular system, it does seem to have the capacity and opportunity to tinker with temperature control. However, much remains to be learned before researchers can say for sure exactly what triggers hot flashes, why some women get them and others don't, why some are more severe than others, and why some women suffer with hot flashes for years while others have them for only a few months.

Estrogen's Effect

Hot flashes drive more women to their doctors for hormone replacement than any other symptom of menopause or any worries about osteoporosis or heart disease. Most of the time the hormones will turn off the heat. "It took effect instantly," announced Madelyn, a New York school teacher whose hot flashes began when she was forty-seven and still having regular periods. "I was miserable. The flashes were unbearable, and I was so depressed that I would go into the ladies room at school, sit on the toilet and cry. I went from doctor to doctor until I found someone willing to put me on hormone replacement."

"I held out for a year," says Jackie, a laboratory manager at a suburban Philadelphia hospital. "By then I was on my knees begging for help. It was physically too tough. I didn't need a winter coat." Jackie's initial inclination to get through menopause without hormone replacement stems from her reluctance to "interfere with nature." Her doctor has told her that she should continue to take hormones for the rest of her life. "We'll see about that," says the still skeptical Jackie.

At sixty, Joy looks, maybe, like she is pushing forty-two. She is ebullient, outgoing, glamorous in the flamboyant Joan Collins mold, and justifiably proud of her slim, muscular body. "I didn't think twice about going topless on the beach when I was in the Caribbean last winter," she laughs, flashing a photo to prove it. A self-described "health nut," Joy works out daily and religiously adheres to a low-fat diet. None of that saved her from several "very rough" years after she reached menopause at fifty-five. "I can understand why women decide to take hormones," says Joy. "If I were still working in an office instead of at home, I might have done it myself. The hot flashes were terrible. I would wake up in a pool of sweat." Her gynecologist urged her to begin hormone replacement, but when Joy asked about the risks, replied only "we'll monitor you."

"That is unacceptable," Joy told me when she described the conversation. "I'm so health oriented, I would rather find a way to muddle through."

Doing Without Estrogen

Unfortunately, muddling through is the only alternative to hormone replacement therapy for hot flashes. Doctors have nothing much to offer apart from a few drugs that don't work dependably and present their own set of risks. Vitamin E, ginseng, and herbal remedies also have their adherents, but none work reliably. Here is a rundown of the available alternatives to estrogen replacement:

• **Clonidine** Clonidine is a drug used to control high blood pressure and, sometimes, to prevent migraine headaches or treat menstrual cramps. The brand name is Catapres or Catapres-TTS. Common (and they *are* common) side effects include fatigue, dry mouth, and extremely vivid dreams. The recommended dose for hot flashes is 0.1–0.2 mg twice a day, much less than the twice daily doses of 0.2–0.8 mg usually taken for high blood pressure. Because it has such unpleasant side effects, clonidine is falling out of favor as a treatment for high blood pressure. Doctors reluctant to prescribe it for a serious medical condition may be even more resistant to prescribing it for hot flashes.

• **Bellergal** Bellergal, a drug for the prevention for migraine headaches, contains ergotamine, phenobarbital (a barbiturate), and caffeine. The most frequent side effect is cold hands and feet with mild numbness and tingling. Less often, Bellergal can cause headache, drowsiness, dizziness, and confusion. Although it *can* relieve or reduce hot flashes, it doesn't always work.

• **Progestin** Treatment with this synthetic form of progesterone can suppress hot flashes. The principal side effect here is uterine bleeding. Although progestin is not approved by the FDA for treatment of menopausal symptoms, doctors can prescribe it to relieve flashes.

• **Vitamin E** Often recommended as a nondrug treatment for hot flashes, vitamin E seems to work for about half of all women who try it although no one knows why. And while it is always high on the list of alternatives to hormone replacement for hot flashes, no studies have verified these claims or looked into the mechanisms by which vitamin E might act to ease or eliminate hot flashes.

A number of researchers have studied the effect of vitamin E on premenstrual syndrome (PMS), but results have been conflicting. If PMS were associated with lower than normal estrogen levels, the fact that vitamin E helps relieve symptoms might provide a clue to why it sometimes works for women with hot flashes. But, in fact, no hormonal differences have ever been found between women with PMS (even those with severe problems) and women who are not affected. And there is no similarity between vitamin E and estrogen.

If you decide to try vitamin E to combat hot flashes, don't expect immediate relief. It can take a month or more for effects to show up. It is best to take vitamin E in divided doses after a meal that includes some fat. You also may have to take 1200 international units (IU) or more per day before you get results.

Vitamin E is considered safe even at high doses. A 1988 study published in the *American Journal of Clinical Nutrition* found "few side-effects to [vitamin E intake] even at doses as high as 3200 IU." However, at 600 IU triglyceride levels increased among some of the women. Other studies have reported side effects ranging from breast soreness (among young women taking 400 to 800 IU) to depression and mood swings among women taking 800 IU. Fatigue, gastrointestinal symptoms, and muscle weakness also have been reported at various dosages.

• **Ginseng** These Chinese herbs (there is more than one type of ginseng) are often recommended for hot flashes. Here, too, you will find no scientific studies in Western medical literature to confirm or refute claims that ginseng effectively relieves hot flashes. However, ginseng does seem to have an estrogenlike effect, so there may be some logic to its reported usefulness. If it does act like estrogen, it would be nice to have some more information about it and the way it affects the body. In their 1977 book *Women and the Crisis in Sex Hormones*, Barbara Seaman and Gideon Seaman, M.D., report that the Chinese, who have been using ginseng medicinally for more than 3000 years, do not do the same kind of scientific studies we do, so all we have to go on here is anecdotal evidence. The bottom line is this: no one has looked at ginseng as rigorously as we expect a substance that acts like a drug to be studied.

If ginseng does have estrogenlike effects, could using it for hot flashes expose you to some of the risks estrogen replacement presents? This is the kind of question you need a well-designed scientific study to answer. It also would be nice to know how much estrogen, if any, you get when you take ginseng capsules or drink ginseng teas. But here, too, we have no information. On the plus side, there have been no published reports that ginseng has had any adverse effects on women who take it for the relief of hot flashes.

If you do decide to take ginseng, you should open up the capsules and use the powder to make tea, advises Kenneth Brown, a consultant to health stores and a fountain of information about natural remedies. Other recommended dosages: one 500 mg tablet twice a day if you weigh less than 130 pounds; one 500 mg tablet three times a day if you weigh up to 160 pounds.

• **Other Natural Remedies** A variety of herbs, alone or in combination, apparently help some women. A product called "Change o' Life" found in some health food stores contains a mixture of these herbs:

- Sarsaparilla
- Black cohosh
- False unicorn
- Blessed thistle
- Squaw vine

One widowed friend in her sixties told me she takes one tablet per day (the recommended dose is six) and that her postmenopausal estrogen levels have increased to the point that her gynecologist was "astonished" and her checkups have been less uncomfortable due to a change for the better in her vaginal tissues.

Ken Brown, my natural remedies guru, tells me that black cohosh (also known as snakeroot and bug wort) is a plant North American Indians used as a treatment for female complaints and rheumatism. It is found in hills at high elevations from Maine to Georgia. There is no scientific evidence that black cohosh works to relieve hot flashes, but *A Friend Indeed,* a menopause newsletter published in Montreal, has carried enthusiastic letters from subscribers who swear by it, and Ken tells me there is a steady demand among his customers.

Black cohosh comes in liquid and tablet form. The liquid extract works fastest. Ken recommends taking 15 drops twice a day. The standard dosage in tablets is 500 mg; Ken advises his customers to take two tablets twice a day at first and increase the dosage until they get relief. Black cohosh does not seem to have a toxic effect so boosting the dosage shouldn't hurt.

Cooling Off

For what it is worth, here is a list of the most frequently recommended strategies for combating hot flashes:
- Avoid coffee and other caffeinated beverages.
- Avoid alcohol.
- Layer your clothing so you can peel off and replace sweaters or jackets.
- Keep a glass of ice water or other cold drink handy.
- Some women say that hot flashes are aggravated by stress, so try to keep your emotional cool.
- Flashes may worsen in hot weather—so park yourself by the air conditioner.

INSOMNIA

Is insomnia a symptom of menopause or a by-product of hot flashes? Since many women awaken during the night to toss off their covers or sop up perspiration from hot flashes, this wakefulness is hard to categorize. However, it is true that many women who do not have hot flashes are troubled by insomnia as they near menopause. It is also important to remember that insomnia is a common problem that often worsens with age.

No one can explain the link between menopause and insomnia. Hormone replacement usually brings relief, and of course, there are all kinds of other remedies you can try, although, if hot flashes are a factor, they probably will continue to wake you. Your doctor may prescribe a sedative like Valium or a sleep aid like the drug Dalmane. Antihistamines that cause drowsiness can help. And then there are the time-tested remedies: a glass of milk (milk contains tryptophan, an amino acid that promotes sleep), a warm bath, a glass of wine, aspirin. Some studies show that regular exercise contributes to a good night's sleep, but I wouldn't count on it. I exercise a lot, and it never had any impact on the sporadic insomnia that has bothered me all my life. And the fact that my friend Joy is still battling the insomnia that arrived with menopause despite her many years of regular exercise makes me even more dubious about claims that it promotes sleep.

DEPRESSION

The stereotype of the menopausal woman as cranky, irritable, moody, depressed, and generally unpleasant company is beginning to yield to yet another stereotype: busy, vital, balanced, and upbeat. Maybe so, but let's face it, cranky, irritable, moody, and depressed are perfectly reasonable and sane responses to hot flashes or insomnia. And busy, vital, balanced, and upbeat may be a little too much to ask under the circumstances. Doesn't menopause entitle women to mix and match moods?

For the record, depression does not seem to be a serious problem for most menopausal women. The biggest study of the subject tracked 2300 Massachusetts women for five years and found that 85 percent reported that they *never* were depressed. About 10 percent appeared to be occasionally depressed and 5 percent persistently depressed, findings that square with the national incidence of depression. Those most likely to suffer were widows, divorcees, and separated women with less than twelve years of education.

Another study, this one from the University of Pittsburgh, followed 541 healthy premenopausal women aged forty-two to fifty to see what psychological effects menopause might have and what symptoms the women would develop. Three years into the study 91 women had reached menopause. Of this number 32 took estrogen. The results showed that natural menopause (without estrogen replacement) did not lead to depression or any of the other negative psychological changes regarded as "classic symptoms" of menopause. In an interview with the *New York Times*, Robert O. Pasnau, a psychiatrist at UCLA Medical School, maintained that "women going through menopause are no more likely to suffer depression than are women at other ages, nor than men for that matter."

If you can't blame menopause for depression, you can probably find the reason elsewhere: an empty nest, aging parents, a husband's midlife crisis, dissatisfaction with your work. And then there is the fact that depression is an epidemic disorder believed to affect one woman in four at some point in life.

Unless depression, irritability, or moodiness stems from hot flashes or insomnia, estrogen replacement won't help, so if depression is a significant problem, you will have to look for the answer elsewhere.

MEMORY LAPSES

Do you keep misplacing your keys, losing your gloves, and forgetting what you meant to do? Many women trace these minor memory lapses to menopause and there is some evidence that estrogen replacement helps. Exactly how diminishing levels of natural estrogen could affect memory isn't known.

JOINT PAIN

Morning stiffness and aches and pains in the joints do seem to be a problem for many women at menopause. These may be related to declining estrogen levels, not just the aging process, since joint pain often occurs regardless of age among women who have had their ovaries removed during hysterectomies. Hormone replacement often relieves these aches and pains. There is also some evidence that hormone replacement lowers the risk of rheumatoid arthritis, a more serious condition than the much more common wear and tear disorder (osteoarthritis) that affects almost everyone sooner or later. And, ominously, aches and pains confined to the back may be early signs of otherwise silent osteoporosis.

SKIN TINGLING

Only a minority of menopausal women develop this weird symptom. They usually describe it as a feeling that insects are crawling on the skin. There is a medical term, *formication*, for this odd problem. No one knows what causes it. Estrogen replacement does seem to help, but even without it the crawly feeling eventually goes away although it can continue for years.

❺ ❺ ❺ ❺

Osteoporosis

DOES MENOPAUSE NECESSARILY mean crumbling bones? Without estrogen are we destined to become stooped old ladies, our backs misshapen by the classic "dowager's hump," the end product of crumbling vertebrae that have become too porous and weak to support the weight of the body? What about the dreaded specter of a broken hip?

Today, estrogen replacement is our best defense against osteoporosis. It slows the rate of bone loss although it won't help replace what already is gone. For best results, treatment should begin within three years of menopause, but even as late as six years after menopause it reduces further loss. Some doctors prescribe estrogen to high-risk women even before menopause occurs.

However, while estrogen replacement can protect against osteoporosis and its disabling and life-threatening consequences, it is no *guarantee* that you won't be affected.

Just how much of a threat does osteoporosis present?

At menopause, all of us are going to begin losing bone. Eventually, this thinning process can lead to osteoporosis. The literal meaning of the word osteoporosis is "porous bones." The threat it presents is huge: according to the National Osteoporosis Foundation a woman's odds of fracturing her hip are equal to the *combined* risk of developing breast, uterine, and ovarian cancer. Being female puts all of us at some risk simply because our bones are smaller than most men's. Bone mass declines with age in both sexes, but being heavier and thicker than women's to start with, men's bones can better withstand the effects of the loss. You can approximate your own risks by looking at your grandmothers, mother, and the other women in your family and by answering the following questions:

1. Are you white? Caucasian women are at higher risk than black women. The extent of the threat to Asian women is unclear. By some estimates one quarter of all white women will have had at least one osteoporosis-related fracture by age sixty-five.

2. Are you petite with small bones?

3. Is your calcium intake low?

4. Do you exercise regularly? Too little exercise can lead to bone loss. On the other hand, women who exercise so much that they cease to menstruate are also at higher than normal risk.

5. Did you reach menopause before age forty-five?

6. Have you had your ovaries removed? If so, your natural estrogen supply has been cut off, placing you at very high risk of osteoporosis. The younger you were at the time of surgery, the higher your risk (unless you have been taking estrogen).

7. Are you underweight? (As far as osteoporosis is concerned, you are better off being overweight. The extra pounds are protective because the weight places stress on the bones causing them to gain strength. Furthermore, because estrogen is produced in fat, over-weight women have higher levels of circulating estrogen. However, being overweight is a mixed blessing: it is a plus for your bones but a minus for your risks of heart disease and breast cancer.)

8. Do you smoke cigarettes? Women who smoke reach meno-pause earlier than nonsmokers. Smoking seems to lower estrogen levels and increases the risk of osteoporosis and bone fractures. Results of a study published in the May 1992 issue of the *Annals of Internal Medicine* showed that estrogen replacement cannot protect you from osteoporosis if you smoke.

9. Are you alcoholic? If so, you are at higher than normal risk for osteoporosis (and many other diseases).

10. Do you take steroid drugs for any medical condition? What about anticoagulants? These drugs will raise your osteoporosis risk.

11. Do you have an overactive thyroid, an overactive parathy-

roid, or kidney disease? All of these will increase your risk of osteoporosis.

Diseases that impair the ability to absorb calcium or a condition called idiopathic hypercalciuria can also pose a threat to your bones.

The more "yes" answers you gave to this little quiz, the higher your risk. Some doctors believe that if you have between four and six of these risk factors you are at high risk of osteoporosis although some risks count more than others. Being white, petite, having a family history of osteoporosis, low calcium intake, and getting little or no regular exercise can be particularly troublesome.

If you consider yourself at high risk, there is little comfort to be found in statistics on the incidence of osteoporosis:

• One third of all American women over fifty eventually will fracture a vertebra. These breaks occur when weakened bone is crushed or compressed by the weight of the body. The fractures usually are painless but sometimes can cause severe back pain. When several vertebrae are crushed, women lose height, and their spines begin to curve.

• Fifteen percent of white women over the age of fifty will fracture their wrists eventually.

• Fifteen percent of white women will fracture a hip.

• All told, osteoporosis affects between 15 and 20 million people in the United States, leads to an estimated 1.3 million fractures per year in people over forty-five, and accounts for about 70 percent of the fractures that occur among this age group. About 1.7 percent of Americans between forty-five and sixty-four and 2 percent of those over sixty-five break a bone because of osteoporosis.

• More than 250,000 osteoporosis-related hip fractures occur every year, three times more often in women than men. Afterward, about half of these people will need some help with daily activities, 15 to 25 percent will need long-term nursing home care, and 12 to 20 percent will die, usually from such complications as pneumonia or blood clots in the lung related to the fracture itself or to surgery required to repair the hip.

BONE BUILDING BASICS

A short course on the formation and structure of bone can help you understand what we're up against. Although our skeletons grow to full size by the late teens, the bones themselves do not reach full density or peak mass until the midthirties. All the while, they are in a constant state of flux, being torn down and rebuilt at the same time. These two processes are known as resorption (tearing down) and remodeling (building up).

Our genes play a role in determining how thick and dense our bones can become. Within this inborn limit the amount of calcium you consume and the extent to which you exercise when you are young determine bone density. Once bone mass reaches its peak in the thirties, the pace of resorption begins to outstrip remodeling and we all begin to lose bone at a slow rate.

There are two types of bone, cortical and trabecular. Cortical bone is the dense, compact layer that forms the outer covering of all bones. Trabecular bone is the porous, spongy inner portion. There is a higher percentage of trabecular bone in the vertebrae and at the ends of the long bones of the arms and legs than elsewhere in the skeleton. Because it is porous to begin with, trabecular bone is particularly susceptible to osteoporosis.

In women, the rate of bone loss that begins in the thirties accelerates at menopause. Declining estrogen levels seem to be responsible although researchers do not have a good grasp of what actually takes place in the body to set this process in motion. However, they have discovered that the cells that build bone (osteoblasts) have receptors for estrogen. This suggests that bone building cells need estrogen to function properly and that without it they may lose some of their effectiveness. (Receptors are small cellular structures often likened to locks that control biochemical access to cells. These "locks" can only be opened by a specific, properly fitting biochemical "key," in this case, estrogen.)

Another biochemical clue to the postmenopausal bone loss is a lessened ability to absorb calcium. Menopausal women also excrete higher than normal levels of calcium in the urine. Exactly how these factors (and others still to be discovered) interact to accelerate bone loss remains a mystery. But there is no doubt about the overall effect: during the three to seven years after menopause, women lose from 2 to 7 percent of bone mass per year! Figure it out: that can amount to almost 50 percent of total bone mass in the first seven years! Most of this loss occurs in the spine. Eventually, the rate of bone loss slows, but it never stops.

If you have strong bones to begin with, if your calcium intake has been high, and if you always have been physically active, you may be able to afford some of this menopausal loss. And if you continue to exercise and get plenty of calcium, you may be able to cut your losses. Most of us aren't in that enviable position and will have to develop a strategy to deal with bone loss.

FIGURING THE ODDS

There is no way to predict accurately the extent of the threat bone loss poses on the basis of risk factors alone. A number of studies have shown that this information failed to predict about 30 percent of all women at high risk for fractures. Robert Lindsay, M.D., director of the Regional Bone Center at the Helen Hayes Hospital in West Haverstraw, New York, and a leading researcher on osteoporosis, emphasizes the need for an objective measurement of bone density should you be considering estrogen replacement. "Just as a physician would not treat you for high blood pressure on the basis of risk factors without taking your blood pressure, you should not decide to take estrogen to protect your bones without some objective quantification of your risk," Lindsay told me in a telephone interview. But not everyone needs testing. An editorial in the October 15, 1990 issue of the *Annals of Internal Medicine* set forth a number of scenarios in which bone density testing would be a waste of time and money:

• When women have had their ovaries removed in the course of hysterectomy. Since they are at *extremely* high risk of both heart disease and osteoporosis, the benefits of estrogen replacement far outweigh the risks.

• When women are principally concerned about preventing heart disease and have already decided to take estrogen.

• When women are unwilling to take hormones under any circumstances.

Today's high-tech, sophisticated tests can provide an assessment of your current bone density and whether it is above or below normal. But they are not accurate enough to predict future fractures. Even women whose bone density is normal or above normal cannot be certain on the basis of test results that their spines won't crumble or that they will not fracture a hip someday. Similarly, women with low bone density cannot be sure that their bones will break if they forego hormone replacement. And since hormone replacement reduces but does not eliminate the risk, even the decision to go this route does not guarantee a fracture-free future. (Incidentally, testing can be expensive, anywhere from $50 to $250 per test depending on where you go.)

Bone Density Tests

Ordinary x-rays used to diagnose fractures cannot detect bone loss until between 25 percent and 40 percent of bone has already disappeared. There is a persistent myth that early signs of osteoporosis will show up on routine dental x-rays. Not true. Bone loss in the jaw doesn't become obvious on dental x-rays until it is well advanced. Better measures of bone density are tests that use photons, units of magnetic energy that are absorbed at a different rate by bone and soft tissue. A technique called photon absorptiometry can determine bone density by measuring the absorption of photons by bones. Some of these tests are so sophisticated that they are available only at research centers and major hospitals, so you may have to do some detective work to find a place to have one.

• **Single Photon Absorptiometry** Single photon absorptiometry measures bone mineral content in the forearm and wrist. Its usefulness is limited because it measures cortical bone not trabecular bone, where osteoporotic losses are most severe.

• **Dual Photon Absorptiometry** Dual photon absorptiometry can measure total cortical and trabecular mineral content of the hip and spine. It takes about twenty minutes.

• **Dual-Energy X-ray Absorptiometry** A newer method, dual-energy x-ray absorptiometry, measures bone density in the hip and spine. It takes only five minutes and provides more precise measurement than dual photon absorptiometry.

• **CAT Scans** CAT scans can measure total bone density or just the density of trabecular bone. However, they are much more expensive than any of the other methods and expose you to a higher dose of radiation. (An average chest x-ray exposes you to more radiation than single or dual photon or dual-energy x-ray absorptiometry.)

• **Quantitative Computed Tomography (QCT)** Quantitative computed tomography, a new computerized analysis of x-ray beams, must be quantified by computer to come up with a measurement of trabecular bone density in the spine.

THE CALCIUM FACTOR

One of the reasons osteoporosis is such a big problem for women is that most of us don't get enough calcium while our bones are growing. If we did, our bones probably would be stronger, and we could better afford the losses we face. Most adult women consume much less than the U.S. recommended dietary allowance (RDA) of calcium, only 450 to 550 milligrams (mg) per day. Some experts believe the RDA of 800 mg a day is too low and that premenopausal women need about 1000 mg of calcium a day. After menopause, women need about 1500 mg of calcium daily to offset losses. If you are typical, you will have to add 1000 mg of calcium a day to your diet to replace the amount you are losing.

Though food is the best calcium source, it is not easy to consume 800 mg daily, let alone the 1500 mg. The table on pages 64, 65, and 66 lists food sources of dietary calcium. Unfortunately, dairy products, the best calcium sources, are also high in saturated fat and calories. If you are watching your weight or following medical recommendations to limit your fat intake, it is tough to get the calcium you need without also consuming calories and fat you are trying to avoid. Notice, however, that skim milk contains more calcium than whole milk or low-fat milk, and that plain, low-fat yogurt will give you more calcium than the same amount of yogurt containing fruit (you can have both if you add fresh fruit to plain yogurt).

Robert Heaney, M.D., an eminent calcium researcher at Creighton University in Omaha, Nebraska, thinks we all would be better off if more food manufacturers fortified their products with calcium. There already are a few on the market. Eight ounces of Citrus Hill Orange Juice provides 300 mg of the 1500 mg you need daily. And one ounce of Total breakfast cereal will give you about 200 mg. If you add one half cup of skim milk to your Total, you'll get an additional 150 mg. If more food manufacturers would add calcium to their products, our problems might be over. But in the meantime, we'll have to find another way. A few hints:

• Although spinach is high in calcium, it isn't a good calcium source because it also contains substances, called oxalates, that interfere with the body's ability to absorb calcium.

• Kale is a great calcium source. When Dr. Heaney conducted a study of this subject, he discovered that of the eleven women who

Some Calcium-Rich Foods

	Measure	Calories	Calcium (mg)
Cheese			
Blue	1 ounce	100	150
Cheddar, cut pieces	1 ounce	115	204
Feta	1 ounce	75	140
Mozzarella, made with whole milk	1 ounce	80	147
Mozzarella, made with part skim milk	1 ounce	80	207
Muenster	1 ounce	105	203
Parmesan	1 tbsp	25	69
Pasteurized process			
American	1 ounce	105	174
Swiss	1 ounce	95	219
Provolone	1 ounce	100	214
Swiss	1 ounce	105	272
Cottage Cheese			
Lowfat (2%)	1 cup	205	155
Creamed (4% fat)			
Large curd	1 cup	235	135
Small curd	1 cup	215	126
Milk			
Skim	1 cup	85	302
1% fat	1 cup	100	300
2% fat	1 cup	120	297
Whole (3.3% fat)	1 cup	150	291
Buttermilk	1 cup	100	285
Dry, nonfat,			
instant	1/4 cup	61	209
Yogurt			
Plain, lowfat, with added milk solids	8 ounces	145	415
Fruit-flavored, lowfat, with added milk			
solids	8 ounces	230*	345*
Plain, whole milk	8 ounces	140	274

*These values may vary.

Some Calcium-Rich Foods (Continued)

	Measure	Calories	Calcium (mg)
Dairy Desserts			
Custard, baked	1 cup	305	297
Ice cream, vanilla Regular (11% fat)			
Hardened	1 cup	270	176
Soft Serve	1 cup	375	236
Ice milk, vanilla			
Hardened, 4% fat	1 cup	185	176
Soft serve, 3% fat	1 cup	225	274
Seafood			
Oysters, raw, meat only (13-19 medium)	1 cup	160	226
Salmon, pink, canned, *including the bones*	3 ounces	120	167**
Sardines, Atlantic, canned in oil, drained, *including the bones*	3 ounces	175	371**
Shrimp, canned, drained, solids	3 ounces	100	98
Vegetables			
Bok choy, raw, chopped	1 cup	9	74
Broccoli, raw	1 spear	40	72
Broccoli, cooked, drained, from raw, ½" pieces	1 cup	45	177
Broccoli, cooked, drained, from frozen, chopped	1 cup	50	94
Collards, cooked, drained, from frozen	1 cup	60	357
Dandelion greens, cooked, drained	1 cup	35	147
Kale, cooked, drained, from frozen	1 cup	40	179
Mustard greens, without stems and mid-ribs, cooked, drained	1 cup	20	104
Turnip greens, chopped, cooked, drained, from frozen	1 cup	50	249
Dried Beans			
Cooked, drained			
Great Northern	1 cup	210	90
Navy	1 cup	225	95
Pinto	1 cup	265	86

**If the bones are discarded, the amount of calcium is greatly reduced.

Some Calcium-Rich Foods (Continued)

	Measure	Calories	Calcium (mg)
Chickpeas (garbanzos), cooked, drained	1 cup	270	**80**
Red kidney, canned	1 cup	230	**74**
Refried beans, canned	1 cup	295	**141**
Soy beans, cooked, drained	1 cup	235	**131**
Miscellaneous			
Molasses, cane, blackstrap	2 tbsp	85	**274**
Tofu, 2 ½" x 2 ¾" x 1" (about 4 ounces)	1 piece	85*	**108***

*Both of these values may vary, especially the calcium content, depending on how the tofu is made. Tofu processed with calcium salts can have as much as 300 mg calcium per 4 ounces. The label, your grocer, or the manufacturer can provide more specific information.

Source: Home and Garden Bulletin #72, Human Nutrition Information Service, U.S. Department of Agriculture, 1985.

participated, nine absorbed the calcium from kale even better than the calcium from milk!

• You will absorb calcium better if you eat the food that contains it along with something else.

• Watch your caffeine consumption: it prompts calcium excretion. A study published in the October 1990 issue of the *American Journal of Epidemiology* showed that individuals who drink more than two cups of coffee or four cups of tea per day increased their risk of hip fracture by 53 percent.

Supplements

If you can't get enough calcium from foods, you will need supplements. Unfortunately, not all calcium supplements are alike. To get the most out of your supplement find one that is high in elemental calcium (this information should be on the label). Calcium carbonate typically contains about 40 percent elemental calcium; calcium lactate 13 percent, and calcium gluconate 9 percent. Most antacids provide calcium carbonate but they also contain aluminum, which can interfere with your ability to absorb calcium from food.

You should also make sure that your supplement is capable of

Nutrients and Substances That Can Enhance or Interfere With Calcium Absorption*

Enhances Calcium Absorption:	
Nutrient/Substance	**Source**
Vitamin D (400 IU)[†]	Egg yolk, salt-water fish, liver, vitamin-D fortified milk
Lactose	Milk
Interferes With Calcium Absorption:	
Substance	**Source**
Oxalates[‡]	Spinach, beets, parsley, rhubarb, summer squash, peanuts, tea, cocoa
Phytates[‡]	Legumes, possibly wheat bran
Fiber[§]	Fruit, vegetables, whole grain bread, cereal products, bran

* In addition to this list, there are nutrients and substances that can cause calcium loss by increasing excretion of calcium in the urine, such as excessive amounts of protein, sodium, or caffeine in the diet.
† USRDA for Vitamin D.
‡ Oxalates and phytates combine with calcium in the intestine to form insoluble complexes that cannot be absorbed. For most people, oxalates and phytates do not interfere seriously with the amount of calcium absorbed. However, in poorly nourished individuals, or those on a high-insoluble-fiber diet (eg, wheat bran), these substances can pose a problem.
§ Consumed in moderation as part of a well-balanced diet, fiber does not significantly interfere with calcium absorption. However, a very high-fiber diet can cause a reduction in calcium absorption especially in certain individuals, such as older persons and the poorly nourished.

Source: National Osteoporosis Foundation, *Boning Up on Osteoporosis,* 1991.

dissolving in your stomach. If it isn't, you won't get any calcium at all. You don't have to worry about this if the container bears a stamp reading "USP Approved," an indication that the brand has met standards set by the U.S. Pharmacopeia. Dr. Heaney told me that, in general, major national brands dissolve far better than drugstore "house" brands or calcium sold in health food stores. However, if you are already using a supplement with no "USP Approved" stamp, you can test it to determine how well it will dissolve in your stomach. Place a tablet in six ounces of vinegar and stir occasionally. If it doesn't disintegrate within thirty minutes, chances are it won't dissolve in your stomach.

Common Calcium Supplement

Form	% Elemental Calcium
Calcium Carbonate	40
Calcium Phosphate (tribasic)	39
Calcium Phosphate (dibasic)	30
Calcium Citrate	21
Calcium Lactate	13
Calcium Gluconate	9

Source: National Osteoporosis Foundation, *Boning Up on Osteoporosis,* 1991.

THE EXERCISE EQUATION

The less physically active you are, the higher your risk of osteoporosis. A long illness that keeps you immobile can result in rapid loss of bone. Even weightlessness in outer space presents problems. Astronauts who have spent time on the Skylab space station and Soviet cosmonauts who lived on space stations lost bone from the heel, hip, and spine. The more time spent away from the earth's gravitational pull, the greater their bone loss. NASA is studying this phenomenon with a view toward preventing it. The results could help us all, but for the time being, the more weight-bearing exercise you get, the stronger your bones are likely to become. With the exception of swimming and yoga, most forms of exercise are weight-bearing. But for the record, here's a list:

- Walking, racewalking, hiking
- Jogging, running
- Jumping rope
- Aerobic dancing
- Ballroom dancing
- Gymnastics
- Tennis, racquetball, squash, handball
- Rowing, weight training
- Basketball, volleyball
- Cross-country skiing

The trouble is no one knows exactly what kind of exercise and how much of it you need to prevent osteoporosis. But it does appear that every little bit helps. A daily walk is a good way to start. However, if you want to try something more strenuous, check with your doctor first, particularly if you are not accustomed to exercise. As I mentioned earlier, too much exercise can be as bad as too little. Women who exercise so much that they stop menstruating may be putting themselves at high risk of osteoporosis. Here, the problem seems to be related to the low levels of body fat. The lower the percentage of fat in your body, the less estrogen you produce. Eventually, estrogen levels fall so low that menstruation ceases. This may be nature's way of announcing that the body is too low on fat to successfully support a pregnancy. Since we need estrogen for bone maintenance, it is vital to keep our reproductive systems in working order for as long as they are capable of functioning.

STRATEGIES TO CONSIDER

Short of estrogen replacement, what can you do to protect your bones? Researchers have come up with some interesting possibilities. Increasing calcium intake may slow the rate of loss *if you also exercise.* Raising calcium intake to 1500 mg and taking a very low dose of estrogen may work as well as traditional hormone replacement therapy. And, if you are more than six years past menopause, there is evidence that taking calcium supplements will cut your rate of bone loss. Here is a rundown of the most promising findings:

• An intriguing study from Australia compared the effects on bone of exercise alone, exercise plus a daily calcium supplement, and exercise plus hormone replacement. A total of 172 women were recruited and divided into three groups. Each group met weekly for an hour-long low impact aerobics class supervised by a trained physical therapist. About twenty minutes of each class was devoted to arm exercises. The women also took two brisk half-hour walks per week. Those in the exercise-calcium group took 1 gram of calcium lactate gluconate per day. Those in the exercise-hormone replacement group took estrogen plus progestin for the duration of the two-year study.

Not surprisingly, hormone replacement plus exercise was the most effective strategy: bone mass *increased* among the women on this regimen. Exercise alone proved useless: the women in this group lost about 2.7 percent of their bone mass, the same amount lost by women in a control group who did not exercise or take calcium or estrogen. The big surprise was that the women who exercised and took calcium lost only half as much bone as those in the control group and those in the exercise-only group.

• Another study, reported in 1987 by Bruce Ettinger, M.D., and a group of researchers at the Kaiser Permanent Medical Center in San Francisco, suggested that a combination of a low dose of estrogen (only 0.3 mg, compared with the standard dose of .625 mg) plus 1500 mg of calcium per day can prevent bone loss. After two years, there was no change in the bone density in the wrists and spines of the women participating. Ettinger and his team also followed a group of women who increased their calcium intake to 1500 mg but did not take any estrogen and a group that opted for no treatment at all. The women in both of these groups lost bone density. A number of other researchers have tried without success to duplicate Ettinger's results, so it is not clear that low-dose estrogen plus calcium is the answer. Still, it might be worth a try although you would need a bone density test before you begin and another after a year or two to find out whether the strategy is working.

• Results of a two-year study at Tufts University, reported in 1990, suggest that calcium supplements can reduce bone loss among women six or more years past menopause. For this study the researchers divided 361 women into two groups: one group took supplements of 500 mg of elemental calcium carbonate or calcium citrate malate; the other took a placebo. At the end of the two years bone density tests showed that the calcium supplements slowed bone loss *only* among women who were six years or more past menopause.

AVAILABLE TREATMENTS AND NEW APPROACHES

Only one drug other than estrogen is available today for treatment of osteoporosis. This substance, salmon-calcitonin, a synthetic form of calcitonin, is a thyroid hormone that inhibits bone resorption (the tear-down process). Although it slows bone loss, salmon calcitonin is not an ideal drug. It must be given by injection, which makes it both inconvenient and expensive (more than $2000 per year), and it can cause a number of very unpleasant side effects: flushing, nausea, vomiting, diarrhea, and abdominal cramps. Because of these limitations, calcitonin treatment is usually reserved for women who are fifteen or more years past menopause and those who cannot take estrogen because of a personal or family history of breast cancer.

A number of other drugs to prevent and treat osteoporosis are under study. They include:

• *Nasal spray calcitonin:* This is calcitonin delivered by nasal spray rather than by injection. It is already being used in Europe but has not been approved in the United States. Although studies have shown that nasal spray calcitonin can prevent early postmenopausal bone loss, there is some question about whether it is fully protective. One study found that it prevents bone loss from the spine but not the forearm.

• *Etridronate (Didronel):* There was a lot of excitement about this drug after the *New England Journal of Medicine* published a study on July 12, 1990, showing that Didronel could strengthen bone and reduce the risk of spinal fractures. Unfortunately, followup studies showed that women who took Didronel suffered a higher rate of fractures than those who were not treated. However, researchers are continuing to study it and similar chemical compounds (bisphosphonates) that may help prevent or treat osteoporosis by inhibiting bone resorption and aiding bone formation.

• *Sodium fluoride:* This compound increases bone mass by stimulating bone building cells, particularly those in trabecular bone. Some studies have found that it reduces the risk of vertebral fractures, but there is also evidence that the bone that grows in response to sodium fluoride is weak and that treatment may lead to an increase in hip fractures. Another drawback is that about 30 percent of all those treated do not respond to the drug at all. Sodium fluoride also causes some unpleasant side effects: 20 to 30 percent of all patients experience nausea, vomiting, and gastrointestinal pain, and up to 40 percent report pain and tenderness in the heels, ankles, and, less often, knees and hips.

• *Thiazide diuretics:* Thiazide diuretics, used to treat high blood pressure, may protect against hip fractures. A study published in the January 15, 1991 issue of the *Journal of the American Medical Association* showed that recent and long-term use is most protective. No effect was seen from past use, and the researchers reported that combination drugs containing thiazides offered no protection.

• *Vitamin D compounds:* Vitamin D compounds look like the most promising drugs on the horizon. One, calcitriol (not to be confused with calcitonin), is an active form of vitamin D. These compounds are widely used to treat osteoporosis in Japan, Italy, New Zealand, and Australia. Hector DeLuca, Ph.D., a vitamin D researcher at the University of Wisconsin, describes calcitriol as a "very potent" drug that not only protects against bone loss but also seems to replace lost bone. A recent study of calcitriol's effect on postmenopausal osteoporosis showed that it significantly reduces the rate of new vertebral fractures. The researchers, a team headed by Murray W. Tilyard, M.D., Ch.B., at the University of Otago in New Zealand, reported their findings in 1992 in the *New England Journal of Medicine.*

The trouble with calcitriol is that it can raise calcium levels so high that a condition called hypercalcemia develops. This, in turn, can (theoretically) lead to kidney stone formation. However, none of the women participating in the New Zealand study ran into any problems, and Dr. Tilyard's team noted that "there is little evidence that the use of calcitriol has ever led to a kidney stone, despite the large number of patients treated."

Dr. DeLuca explained that because of calcitriol's effects on calcium levels, use of the drug in the United States probably would require some physician and patient education. When you take this drug, you have to keep calcium consumption low (just the opposite of what we've been encouraged to do to protect against osteoporosis). The women in the New Zealand study had an average dietary calcium intake of 800 mg and ran into no problems. Still, Dr. Tilyard's team cautioned that blood calcium levels should be monitored in patients taking calcitriol. Calcitriol seems to cause few side effects. The principal one noted during the New Zealand study was nausea, but very few of the women participating were affected.

Meanwhile, Dr. DeLuca and some of his colleagues at the University of Wisconsin have received a patent for a variety of vitamin D called 1-alpha hydroxyvitamin D2. This synthetic substance appears to prevent bone loss without causing excessive calcium buildup. If studies confirm that it works as well as earlier research indicates and no problems with calcium accumulation develop, we could have a powerful new weapon against osteoporosis by 1995.

❻ ❶ ❌

Heart Disease and Women

PERHAPS THE MOST widespread misconception about heart disease is that women don't get it. The truth is that young women rarely get it. However, heart disease is the number one killer of women over sixty, claiming 250,000 lives per year.

We tend to think of heart disease as a male problem because it can strike men at a relatively young age. One out of every three men under sixty (compared to one in ten women) develops heart disease. Women's risk begins to rise at menopause but does not equal men's until about ten years later. Still, whatever the age, whatever the sex, heart disease remains our number one enemy: every year 1.5 million Americans have heart attacks; 500,000 die, 300,000 of them before they reach the hospital. All told, nearly 5 million Americans have heart disease. Millions more are courting disaster because they have high blood pressure, high cholesterol, or both.

Surprisingly, heart disease is more severe among women over sixty than among men of the same age, and women are twice as likely as men to die within sixty days of suffering a heart attack. Women are also less likely to survive coronary bypass surgery. One possible explanation is that our coronary arteries are smaller than men's, making the operation itself more difficult. Another is that women tend to be older and sicker than men at the time of surgery. It also appears that high triglyceride levels may elevate women's risk of heart disease, while there is no evidence that they have the same effect in men.

A Silent Killer

Heart disease does not develop overnight. It can begin as early as childhood and progress slowly and stealthily for years until the first symptoms appear. This disease process, atherosclerosis, is the slow accumulation of fatty deposits, called atheroma, on the inner linings of major arteries. The deposits consist of cholesterol, cellular wastes, calcium, and fibrin, a blood substance involved in the clotting process. A pile-up, or clump, of atheroma is called plaque. As plaque accumulates, arteries that are normally elastic and supple become rigid and inflexible. The end result is arteriosclerosis, or hardening of the arteries. In time, plaque can become so thickly encrusted that it narrows or blocks the passage through the arteries reducing the free flow of blood toward the heart.

The most dramatic outcome of coronary artery blockage is a heart attack. While the presence of a blockage sets the stage, the most important precipitating factor here is formation of a blood clot (or thrombus) in an artery clogged with plaque. If the clot cannot squeeze through the area of the artery narrowed by plaque, it will act like a plug and prevent blood from flowing past it to the heart. Deprived of the oxygen blood supplies, the heart's regular rhythm goes haywire. The sooner the clot is dissolved, the faster blood flow resumes. Heart attack treatment now relies heavily on clot-dissolving drugs. One way to protect against heart attacks is to take a daily aspirin tablet. Aspirin reduces the tendency of blood constitutents called platelets to stick together and form clots.

Blood flow doesn't have to be blocked to cause heart problems. When the supply is diminished, even temporarily, the heart may not get adequate oxygen. This can result in chest pain (angina pectoris) or silent myocardia ischemia, a painless response to oxygen deprivation. Both are symptoms of coronary artery disease, the potentially fatal outcome of atherosclerosis.

THE FEMALE ADVANTAGE

No one knows exactly what protects premenopausal women against heart disease. One seemingly obvious explanation is the fact that prior to menopause most women have low cholesterol levels. Younger women are also more likely than men of the same age to have high levels of high density lipoprotein (HDL), the "good" cholesterol that protects against heart disease by sweeping artery-clogging fats out of blood vessels. After menopause, HDL levels drop about 4 milligrams per deciliter of blood (mg/dl). At the same time, low density lipoprotein (LDL), the "bad" cholesterol associated with fats that clog arteries, rises 12 mg/dl. These post-menopausal changes in cholesterol levels coupled with the fact that, at the same time, the incidence of heart disease begins to rise suggest that estrogen is responsible for the low rate of heart disease among women of reproductive age. However, surprisingly little research has been done to confirm that estrogen really does account for the low rate of heart disease among young women and, if so, how it operates in the body to achieve this remarkable effect.

Even fewer studies have investigated other factors that might protect young women from heart disease. Conceivably, the number of times a woman has given birth or her menstrual history could influence her risk, but in a 1991 article in the *Journal of the American Medical Association (JAMA)* two prominent researchers, Elizabeth Barrett-Conner, M.D., and Trudy Bush, Ph.D., reported that, so far, no statistically significant associations have been found between the low rate of heart disease in young women and either of these factors. If such a link did exist, it might suggest that a particular hormonal mechanism contributes to the protection young women enjoy.

One intriguing new theory holds that the regular loss of iron in menstrual blood protects premenopausal women. The chief proponent of this view, Jerome L. Sullivan, M.D., Ph.D., a researcher at the Veterans Affairs Medical Center in Charleston, South Carolina, notes that several studies have suggested a link between heart disease and high blood levels of iron. However, so far there is no evidence demonstrating that low iron levels are protective. And, no other possibility has come to light.

THE CASE FOR ESTROGEN REPLACEMENT

For years, researchers have been accumulating evidence that estrogen replacement lowers the risk of heart disease among postmenopausal women. The latest and most impressive data come from the Nurses Health Study being conducted by a team of researchers at a group of hospitals affiliated with Harvard Medical School. Their results, reported in September 1991 in the *New England Journal of Medicine,* showed that women taking estrogen replacement have half the normal risk of heart disease.

When the ten-year study was launched, none of the 48,470 postmenopausal nurses who signed up had a history of heart disease. Half took estrogen and half did not. The results showed that the rate of heart disease among the nurses who took estrogen was half of what it was among the nurses who did not take estrogen.

In their *JAMA* article Drs. Barrett-Connor and Bush estimated that between 25 percent and 50 percent of the protection estrogen replacement affords is due to beneficial changes in HDL and LDL: HDL levels increase while LDL levels decline. But, the two researchers were unable to account for the other 50 percent to 75 percent of the protection. They noted that there is very little information about how estrogen might affect clotting factors in the blood (although they conceded that the few studies that have been done have shown little or no effect). Barrett-Connor and Bush suggested several mechanisms by which estrogen may lower women's risks:

• Maintains blood pressure at normal levels.

• Improves carbohydrate metabolism, which, in turn, would lower blood sugar and insulin levels, both of which can influence the risk of heart disease.

• Advantageously affects levels of several hormones that could otherwise contribute to heart disease.

However, here the two researchers were speculating: no one knows whether estrogen exerts any influence in any of these areas.

THE PROGESTIN CONNECTION

The big question the Nurses Study left unanswered is whether estrogen replacement protects against heart disease when women also take progestin. The nurses took estrogen alone, not the estrogen plus progestin usually prescribed today. (Progestin was not widely prescribed for this purpose until the mid-1980s, nearly ten years after the Nurses Study began.)

A number of studies have suggested that progestin may diminish or cancel out the beneficial effect estrogen has on HDL. If so, taking both hormones would not work as well to lower the risk of heart disease as estrogen alone. We should learn a lot more about progestin's effect in 1994 when results of a three-year study being conducted by the National Heart Lung and Blood Institute become available. This $10 million effort, the Postmenopausal Estrogen/Progestin Interventions Trial (better known as PEPI), is testing the effects of estrogen alone, three estrogen/progestin combinations, and a placebo on (1) cholesterol (including HDL and LDL); (2) blood pressure; (3) fibrinogen; and (4) insulin. The PEPI results also should tell us more about how estrogen protects women against heart disease.

WHAT WE DON'T KNOW

Could the studies showing that estrogen replacement protects against heart disease be wrong? There are medical experts who think so, although these nay-sayers are in the minority. But even Trudy Bush and Elizabeth Barrett-Conner, who maintain that evidence suggesting that estrogen replacement protects women from heart disease is "strong, reasonably consistent and biologically plausible," have expressed some reservations. With one exception all of the data showing that estrogen protects women's hearts come from population studies in which large groups of women are observed. This is not the way drugs are usually evaluated.

The trouble with the population studies is that there is no way to be sure if the women taking estrogen were healthier to start with than the women in the comparison groups. If they were—and they may have been—the results would not be as meaningful. Critics argue that, in general, women who don't take estrogen are twice as likely to be seriously overweight than those who do. Furthermore, women who do not take estrogen are more likely to have high blood pressure or diabetes.

In contrast, women who take estrogen tend to be thinner, more physically active, and more health conscious than those who do not. If this was the case among the women participating in the population studies, the results would be biased to some degree: thin, active, and health conscious women are at low risk of heart disease whether or not they take estrogen.

The critics complain that researchers who conduct big population studies have no idea of the medical reasoning underlying the women's decisions to take—or not take—estrogen. Some of these reasons could be related to health problems that would increase—or decrease—their heart disease risk.

Some other nagging questions have emerged from studies suggesting that estrogen may *increase* the risk of heart disease. One of these involved men who were given estrogen to see if it would protect them as well as it seems to protect women. That study was halted ahead of schedule because the men taking the biggest doses of estrogen developed a much higher than normal rate of heart disease.

And then there is a respected study that showed that women who took estrogen had a *higher* rate of heart disease than those who did not. Those results may have been due to the fact that the women were taking much higher doses of estrogen than commonly prescribed today. (Estrogen's protective effect seems to disappear when the dose exceeds 1.25 mg.)

Concerns about estrogen's effects on the heart also stem from evidence that prolonged use of birth control pills increases the risk of cardiovascular problems. This may not be relevant, since the amount of estrogen in the pill is much higher than the amount prescribed for postmenopausal women. It is also a different type of estrogen.

The only way to answer the estrogen questions definitively would be to compare two groups of women with similar risks. This would require a double-blind, randomized clinical trial in which one group of women would take estrogen and the other a placebo. Writing in the same issue of the *New England Journal of Medicine* that carried the results of the Nurses Study, Lee Goldman, M.D., and Anna N.A. Tosteson, Sc.D., of Brigham and Women's Hospital in Boston, called for a clinical trial to document that the population study results are not a "function of bias or statistical legerdemain." They added that "it is hard to justify the past delay, let alone any future foot-dragging" on such an important matter.

Some of the concerns about estrogen's effect on heart disease risk will be addressed by a massive Women's Health Initiative planned by the National Institutes of Health. Researchers will also look into the effect of estrogen/progestin combinations. But don't expect any news before the turn of the century: the study, scheduled to begin in 1993, will continue for nine years.

ASSESSING YOUR RISKS

To decide whether you need estrogen to protect against heart disease, you need to know as much as possible about your personal risk. The sections that follow will help you determine where you stand.

Weight

For women, the best way to protect against heart disease may be to get thin and stay that way. Results of an eight-year Harvard Medical School study of 115,886 women aged thirty to fifty-five at the outset showed that being even mildly overweight increases the risk of heart disease. After correcting for other pertinent risks such as smoking, drinking alcohol, high blood pressure, diabetes, high cholesterol, menopausal status, family history, and fat and cholesterol consumption, the researchers found that *as much as 70 percent* of the coronary disease observed among obese women could be attributed to weight alone. The other findings are a good argument for weight control:

• Forty percent of coronary disease found among *all* the women was related to excess weight.

• The leanest group of women had the lowest rate of heart disease.

• Women of average weight had risks that were about 30 percent higher than those of the leanest women.

• A weight gain during adulthood *doubled* a woman's risk.

This study did not take into consideration earlier research suggesting that obesity increases the risk of heart disease only when fat is concentrated in the abdomen (the classic beer belly more typical of men than women). However, the researchers noted that "if any one aspect of obesity is related more specifically to coronary disease," their results would *underestimate* the magnitude of the problem. This means that if you are overweight and your excess pounds are concentrated in your abdomen, your risk of heart disease is even higher than the Harvard study results suggest! If it isn't obvious in the mirror, a quick way to determine where your weight is concentrated

Desirable Weights* for Women (Ages 25 and Over)

Height†		Small	Medium	Large
Feet	Inches	Frame	Frame	Frame
4	10	92–98	96–107	104–119
4	11	94–101	98–110	106–122
5	0	96–104	101–113	109–125
5	1	99–107	104–116	112–128
5	2	102–110	107–119	115–131
5	3	105–113	110–122	118–134
5	4	108–116	113–126	121–138
5	5	111–119	116–130	125–142
5	6	114–123	120–135	129–146
5	7	118–127	124–139	133–150
5	8	122–131	128–143	137–154
5	9	126–135	132–147	141–158
5	10	130–140	136–151	145–163
5	11	134–144	140–155	149–168
6	0	138–148	144–159	153–173

* Weight in pounds according to frame (indoor clothing).
† With 1-inch heel shoes on for men and 2-inch heel shoes on for women.

Source: Metropolitan Life Insurance Company Actuarial Tables, 1959.

is to measure your waist and hips. A woman's waist should measure no more than 80 percent of her hips. (A man's waist should be no larger than his hips.)

While there is some controversy about what actually constitutes ideal or desirable weight, most experts accept the Metropolitan Life Insurance Company height/weight tables published in 1959 as the most reliable guide to healthy weight.

The Cholesterol Connection

Your cholesterol level is determined partly by heredity and partly by diet (meats, dairy products, and other foods from animal sources contain cholesterol; fruits, vegetables, and grains do not). In the bloodstream, cholesterol travels in tiny spherical packets called lipoproteins composed of cholesterol itself (a lipid or fat) and protein. Low density lipoprotein (LDL) is associated with damage to blood vessels that leads to heart disease. The higher your LDL, the greater your risk. High density lipoprotein (HDL) carries cholesterol out of the bloodstream and back to the liver where it is processed for elimination from the body. The higher your HDL, the lower your risk.

Many of the factors that increase the risk of heart disease itself also influence cholesterol levels:

• Diet: The more foods you eat containing saturated fats, the higher your cholesterol is likely to be. (Animal products are the main sources of saturated fat.)

• Weight: Every extra two pounds contributes 1 milligram of cholesterol per deciliter (one tenth of a liter) of blood.

• Inactivity: Lack of exercise is related to low levels of HDL, the "good" cholesterol.

• Alcohol: Moderate drinking may increase HDL.

• Stress: Although some studies have suggested that stress raises cholesterol levels, stress also prompts many people to overeat, so the cholesterol increase may be food-related.

CHOLESTEROL: WHAT THE NUMBERS MEAN

Here's how doctors rate cholesterol levels:
  • *Desirable:* under 200
  • *Borderline:* 200–240
  • *High risk:* more than 240

A lipid analysis (a laboratory test done on a blood sample drawn after an overnight fast) determines HDL, LDL, and triglyceride levels. The higher your LDL, the higher your risk:
  • *Desirable:* below 130
  • *Borderline high risk:* 130–159
  • *High risk:* above 160

The higher your HDL, the lower your heart disease risk:
  • *Low risk:* more than 70
  • *Average risk:* 35–70
  • *High risk:* below 35

Triglycerides

Normal triglyceride levels range from about 50 to 250 mg/dl. A triglyceride level between 250 and 500 constitutes a "borderline elevation" that may increase heart disease risk in women (this is less significant among men).

High Blood Pressure

Women are less likely than men to develop high blood pressure and, mysteriously, we can tolerate higher levels without adverse effects. However, that doesn't mean that we are not at risk for heart attack and stroke when high blood pressure is uncontrolled.

Blood pressure is considered normal unless it exceeds 140/90. However, for women there usually is no cause for concern as long as pressure is below 160/95.

No one knows what causes high blood pressure. At one time, it appeared that salt intake was to blame, since high blood pressure is rare among people who don't consume much salt. However, it turns out that the salt factor does not apply to everyone: less than 10 percent of all people are salt-sensitive (if you are salt-sensitive your blood pressure rises in response to the amount of salt you consume). Since there's no easy way to determine who is salt-sensitive and who is not, doctors usually urge everyone with high blood pressure to limit salt intake.

Weight also influences blood pressure: about 60 percent of all hypertensives are overweight; if you are 30 percent or more overweight, you are twice as likely to develop high blood pressure as someone of normal weight. Sometimes losing weight is all the treatment needed.

Smoking

Cigarette smoking not only increases the risk of heart disease it multiplies the dangers posed by high blood pressure or high cholesterol. The risk of heart disease begins to drop as soon as you stop smoking and ten years later will be no greater than if you never smoked.

Heredity

The hereditary risk of heart disease is greatest when a parent, brother, or sister develops heart disease or dies of a heart attack before age 55. A strong pattern of early deaths suggests that some genetic defect is being passed from one generation to the next. One such defect disturbs the way the body handles cholesterol. However, even these inborn risks can be overcome: when affected families look back a few generations, they often find that grandparents or great-grandparents lived well into their sixties and seventies, an indication that the more active lives and healthier diets that prevailed in the not-so-distant past were powerful enough to overcome a genetic predisposition to heart disease.

Lack of Exercise

Even moderate exercise can lower the risk of premature death from heart disease. A daily walk of a half-hour or an hour is enough to improve the odds. A twenty-four-week study at the Cooper Institute for Aerobics Research in Dallas, Texas, showed that women who walk three miles a day five days a week can reduce their risk of heart disease regardless of how fast they walk. The study found that women who walked a mile in twelve minutes and those who did it in twenty minutes had the same advantageous 6 percent increase in HDL. (None of the women lost weight but they did decrease their percentage of body fat.)

Earlier studies have found that heart disease risks are lowest among women who exercise strenuously enough to burn 2000 calories per week with exercise. However, exercise does not cancel out the harmful effects of smoking.

Stress and Personality

Stress is often related to the amount of control we have over our lives—the more control, the less stress. Heart disease is more common among people in jobs that entail a great deal of responsibility but little or no control: inner-city high school teachers, police officers, miners, air-traffic controllers, medical interns, stockbrokers, journalists, people who work in customer service or complaint departments, waitresses, and secretaries.

The notion that personality contributes to heart disease comes from a study published in 1959 indicating that hard-driving, aggressive, and hostile (Type A) men are affected twice as often as more easygoing (Type B) individuals. However, more recent findings indicate that Type A behavior may be more of a help than a hazard to people with heart disease. One study showed that among heart attack victims who lived beyond the first critical twenty-four hours, the death rate was notably lower among the Type As!

Diabetes

An estimated 10 million Americans are diabetic, but at least half of those affected don't know it. Because diabetes can be life-threatening, if you are seriously overweight, you should have your blood sugar checked every year. Diabetics have twice the normal risk of heart disease. Diet and exercise or, in more severe cases, insulin, can control diabetes but the risk of heart disease remains abnormally high.

SEVEN

Breast Cancer

THE BIG QUESTION surrounding estrogen replacement is whether or not it can lead to breast cancer. The short answer here is unsatisfactory: it can, but the risk does not seem to be very high. The long answer is much more complex. Every time a study shows a slight increase in breast cancer risk with estrogen replacement, researchers remind us that, statistically, heart disease presents a far greater threat and that, on balance, the benefits of taking estrogen far outweigh the relatively small risk.

That is small comfort if you have a family history of breast cancer, or, like many women, you fear breast cancer more than heart disease or crumbling bones. Some of us almost certainly should worry more about heart disease and/or osteoporosis than the apparently small added risk of breast cancer presented by estrogen replacement.

Based on the best information available today the breast cancer risk among women taking estrogen is small and confined to those who have been on hormone replacement for ten years or more. How small? The increased risk is about 40 percent. This sounds worse than it is. What it means is that at age sixty when one woman in every 420 gets breast cancer, one in every 300 women taking estrogen will develop the disease.

Those are reassuring numbers, but much more remains to be learned about the risk. Today, concern is focused on the added breast cancer threat posed by taking progestin as well as estrogen. Progestin has been widely used only since the mid-1980s, so it may be too soon to see an effect. And then there is the fact that this question simply has not yet been extensively studied.

The breast cancer issue is so emotionally loaded that your peace of mind may be threatened by any added risk. Breast cancer is all around us. Lately, it seems that not a month goes by without news that yet another friend or friend of a friend has just been diagnosed. Given the fact that the incidence of the disease rises with age, you may have come to the justifiable conclusion that your risks are already high enough and getting higher every day, estrogen or no estrogen. But since estrogen is the best defense we have against osteoporosis and the only reliably effective treatment for the symptoms of menopause, you may feel more comfortable about the risks it poses after evaluating your odds of developing breast cancer.

WHAT THE STUDIES SHOW

If you want to believe that estrogen does NOT cause breast cancer, you can find plenty of comforting data among the many studies of the subject. And if you read the medical literature, you will see that well-intentioned, respected experts differ profoundly in the way they interpret the data. The pivotal study on the breast cancer–estrogen replacement question was conducted by Lief Bergkvist, M.D., and a research team at the University Hospital in Uppsala, Sweden. Results were published in 1989 in the *New England Journal of Medicine*. Dr. Bergkvist assessed the effects of estrogen plus progestin on breast cancer risk. He found that among a group of women who took both drugs the breast cancer rate was four times as high as normal. However, since relatively few Swedish women participating in the study took progestin in combination with estrogen for a number of years, the researchers said they could not be certain that the increased risk seen is meaningful. Among the women who took estrogen alone, the rate of breast cancer was twice that of women who took no hormones.

Although the Swedish study was hailed as a "landmark" when it was published, critics came forward almost immediately to take issue with the results and argue that they cannot be applied to

American women. In the first place, most of the women participating in the Swedish study took estradiol, a very potent form of estrogen not prescribed in the United States. Dr. Bergkvist emphasized this difference in the report on his study and conceded that there was no "clear evidence of an increased risk of breast cancer after the use of conjugated estrogens," the type most commonly used in the United States.

Some critics of the Swedish findings have questioned whether they really reflect an increased risk of breast cancer or just the effects of early detection of cancer, since women who take estrogen usually are screened for breast cancer with both physical examinations and mammography. If the women in the comparison group did not have physical exams and mammograms, they may have had an amount of undetected cancer equal to the increased incidence seen among the estrogen users.

Despite the medical debate it stimulated, the Swedish study is important, and its findings cannot be dismissed. A year later, a prestigious group of researchers associated with the Harvard School of Public Health published the results of a ten-year study that showed a 30 to 40 percent increase in the risk of breast cancer among women taking estrogen. The researchers allowed for the difference in breast cancer incidence that might be due to early detection and found that the increased risk of cancer was real, not a reflection of early diagnosis. They found no association between the dose of estrogen women took and their risk of cancer. The best news this study produced was that once a woman stops using estrogen her increased breast cancer risk returns to normal.

Earlier studies of the breast cancer–estrogen connection were much more reassuring. Most showed no increased risk at all, and some actually suggested that estrogen protects women: they found less cancer among the estrogen users than among the comparison groups. Today, most researchers give more credence to the newer studies and agree that estrogen replacement does increase a woman's risk of breast cancer and that the risk may be higher still when a woman takes progestin as well as estrogen.

ESTROGEN AND THE BREAST

It is not surprising that estrogen should be associated with an increased risk of breast cancer. Researchers have long known that the longer a woman is exposed to estrogen, the higher her breast cancer risk. Forget about estrogen replacement for a moment and consider the estrogen we all produce naturally. Observations of who gets breast cancer and who doesn't suggest that the longer our bodies are exposed to estrogen, the higher the risk of developing breast cancer. For instance, women who start menstruating early and stop late are at higher risk, particularly if they menstruate for more than forty years. On the other hand, women whose primary estrogen supply is cut off when their ovaries are removed during a hysterectomy before they reach menopause have a lower rate of breast cancer. The presence or absence of estrogen is the common thread here.

And then there is the fact that most breast cancers that develop among postmenopausal women are estrogen dependent—that is, they need estrogen to grow. A test performed during the biopsy of a malignant lump can show whether the tumor cells are equipped with estrogen receptors, tiny structures usually described as locks that control access to the cells. Receptors are specific to a single body chemical, the only key that can fit the lock. Thus, an estrogen receptor is like a lock that can be opened only by estrogen. When breast cancer is diagnosed, treatment will depend on whether it is estrogen dependent. If it is, doctors often will prescribe tamoxifen, a synthetic hormone that jams the receptors so they no longer can be unlocked by estrogen.

BREAST CANCER

You probably know the statistics: one out of nine women will develop breast cancer in her lifetime. The incidence of the disease has been increasing at an alarming rate, up 32 percent between 1982 and 1987 (the last year for which complete figures are available). No one knows why the rate of breast cancer is rising so fast, although some doctors suspect that early diagnosis via mammograms is responsible. Because more women are having mammograms, more early breast cancers may be turning up, but most experts agree that this doesn't fully explain the increase. In all likelihood, environmental influences not yet identified are to blame. In this context "environmental" does not necessarily mean pollution or carcinogens. Used in a scientific sense, it refers to everything that happens to us after conception—that is, after the genetic input is complete.

This includes our diets and whether or not we drink alcohol, as well as any other outside influences on health (including whether—and for how long—we took birth control pills and/or estrogen replacement). With a few notable exceptions—cigarette smoking, exposure to asbestos, or the sun—it is difficult, if not impossible, to pinpoint the cause of any kind of cancer. For instance, we know that cigarette smoking can lead to lung cancer, although no one can predict which smokers will get sick and which ones won't.

Researchers suspect that some people are born with a vulnerability to cancer. If so, this genetic predisposition is not necessarily destiny. Another event usually must take place to trigger the biological process that leads to cancer. In the case of breast cancer, a number of possible "triggers" have been identified.

ASSESSING YOUR RISKS

The strongest risk factor for breast cancer is a family history, but 70 percent of all women who develop the disease have no affected relatives. In order to establish your personal risks you have to consider all of the known risk factors and determine how many affect you. But first you should know something about how risk is measured. The fact that one woman in nine will develop breast cancer is correct but somewhat deceptive. It is a statement of lifetime risk and tells us how many women will develop breast cancer at some point in their lives, not how many will get it this year.

More to the point is the concept "relative" risk, the additional risks (if any) that pertain to you as compared with women who have no such risks. The difference is the *relative* risk. Since just being female puts all of us at some risk, normal risk is always stated as one. Thus, if you look at the total number of women at, say, age fifty (see the table on 93) who can expect to develop breast cancer, you will see that it works out to one in every 49. If you have twice the normal risk, you have two chances in 49 of developing cancer (not two chances out of nine). If you have ten times the normal risk, your odds are ten in 49 and so on.

The breast cancer risk most of us focus on is family history, but there are a number of others that come into play. If no woman in your family has had breast cancer, you may want to skip the sections below and turn to 94 to read about the other risks.

FAMILY HISTORY

If your mother had breast cancer, your own risk is higher than normal. How high it is depends on whether any of your other relatives are affected and, if so, how many. The fact that breast cancer runs in some families suggests that some type of mutation or damage to a gene may be responsible.

In 1990 a research team at Massachusetts General Hospital identified a defect in a gene that normally helps suppress tumor growth and appears to predispose to breast cancer and a number of other cancers. Anyone born with this genetic defect has an extraordinarily high cancer risk, but, so far, the defect has been seen only in families suffering from a very rare disorder, Li-Fraumeni syndrome, in which close relatives suffer from one or more types of cancer. The women in these families usually develop breast cancer and the men tend toward cancers of the brain, blood, muscle, bone, bone marrow, and adrenal gland. Apart from this new discovery, medical researchers know that breast cancer falls into three distinct categories: sporadic, familial, and hereditary.

Sporadic Breast Cancer

More than 70 percent of women who develop breast cancer come from families with no trace of the disease through two generations when everyone can be accounted for: both sets of grandparents, parents, aunts, uncles, brothers, sisters, and all their children.

There is no way to predict what these "sporadic" cancers mean to future generations. If the cancer stems from a mutation in a gene that the affected woman already has passed along to her daughters, they, too, would be susceptible. Most of the time, however, sporadic breast cancer appears to be a freak of nature in otherwise healthy families. If the victim's daughter eventually develops breast cancer, there is no way to tell if it is due to a genetic mutation or just rotten luck, given the high rate of breast cancer these days.

Even so, a woman whose mother had breast cancer has twice the normal risk of developing the disease herself. Given that the normal relative risk is one, twice that risk is not as frightening as it sounds. Put in perspective, it means that if the normal chance of developing breast cancer by age fifty is one in 49, a woman whose mother had the disease has a risk of 2.3 in 49. Here is a rundown on the approximation of the risks posed by other breast cancer scenarios:

• A woman with an affected aunt or grandmother: 1.5, only slightly higher than normal.

• A woman with an affected mother *and* sisters: 14 times normal.

• Sisters of women who had cancer in both breasts diagnosed between the ages of forty and fifty: 5 times normal. This rises to 10.5 times higher than normal when the cancer was diagnosed before the affected woman's fortieth birthday.

• Sisters of women who had cancer in only one breast diagnosed between the ages of forty and fifty: NO increased risk.

• Sisters of women with cancer in one breast diagnosed at age forty or younger: 2.4 times higher than normal.

• Women with family histories of breast cancer who have had breast biopsies for benign conditions that revealed atypical hyperplasia, an excess of cells with some abnormal but nonmalignant features in the milk ducts: between 4.4 and 11 times normal.

An optimistic note on this subject came from a 1990 study at Rush-Presbyterian-St. Luke's Hospital in Chicago suggesting that the higher breast cancer risk among women with a positive family history declines with age. The researchers found that odds of developing breast cancer were highest when women with a family history of the disease were between thirty and thirty-four years old. After that, the risks begin to drop and, by the time a woman passes sixty, level off at normal. Just why the risk should decline with age is not known. The results came as such a surprise that they will have to be confirmed by other studies before we can accept them as valid.

Familial Breast Cancer

When two or more first- or second-degree relatives are affected, breast cancer is considered "familial." About 25 percent of all cases fall into this category. Daughters and sisters of women with familial breast cancer have three times the normal risk although when cancer occurs at a very young age—under thirty—the risks could be even higher. The more affected relatives and the younger they are at the time of diagnosis, the more likely it is that the breast cancer is hereditary in nature.

Hereditary Breast Cancer

About 9 percent of all breast cancer is considered hereditary and presents an enormous risk. Affected families have an extraordinary amount of cancer. The following factors suggest that breast cancer is hereditary:

• Cancer occurs in more than one generation and is transmitted from mother or father to daughter. (A man can be a carrier of the tell-tale genetic trait even though he, himself, is unaffected.)

• An unusually early age at onset, typically fifteen to twenty years earlier than age sixty, the average age at which breast cancer occurs; some hereditary breast cancers develop among women in their early and midtwenties.

• Cancer often occurs in both breasts, but not necessarily at the same time.

• Cancer occurs in other sites in the body, often the colon or ovaries.

The only way to determine whether your family fits the hereditary pattern is a careful investigation of the incidence of cancer among all of your relatives going back as many generations as possible. In most cases, there is no way to determine which women in these cancer-prone families are destined to develop the disease and which are not. However, researchers have discovered a biochemical marker for the defective gene responsible for a family propensity to breast and ovarian cancer known as the hereditary breast and ovarian cancer syndrome. Women from these families can now be tested for the presence of the marker. Those who test positive are virtually certain to develop one or both of these diseases and then may choose to protect themselves by having their ovaries and breasts removed.

The risks for women from families with other patterns of hereditary breast cancer may run as high as 50–50. Experts on hereditary cancer often advise women from these families to have their breasts removed prophylactically.

Much of the research on hereditary breast cancer is being carried out by Henry T. Lynch, M.D., of the Hereditary Cancer Institute at Creighton University in Omaha, Nebraska (see Appendix 1 for the institute's address). Dr. Lynch has developed the following guidelines for women in high-risk families:

• Examine your own breasts monthly without fail.

• Begin having mammograms at age twenty-five; have one every other year until you reach thirty-five and then have them annually. If any of your relatives developed breast cancer at a young age, begin having *annual* mammograms five years before the earliest age of diagnosis in your family.

• See your doctor twice a year for a breast examination.

• Learn as much as you can about hereditary breast cancer.

AGE

Less than 10 percent of all cases occur among women under thirty. After that, the rate doubles every five years between the ages of thirty and forty-five and then increases by 10 to 15 percent every five years thereafter.

The table below presents the risk of breast cancer from age 30 to age 85:

Age	Risk
30	one in 2550
40	one in 208
50	one in 49
60	one in 23
70	one in 14
80	one in 10
85	one in 9

Source: American Cancer Society.

FIBROCYSTIC DISEASE

Fibrocystic disease is a meaningless medical catch-all term coined to refer to lumpy, tender breasts. The same goes for two other terms sometimes used to describe this common and harmless problem: chronic cystic mastitis and mammary dysplasia. Half of all women complain of these symptoms at one time or another. Usually, both the lumpiness and tenderness show up premenstrually and disappear after menstruation begins.

Sometimes, radiologists use the term "fibrocystic" to refer to dense breast tissue seen on mammograms, and pathologists may refer to microscopic but harmless changes seen in breast tissue removed during a biopsy as "fibrocystic." In no case does a "fibrocystic" condition increase the risk of breast cancer. However, one benign breast change does elevate the cancer risk.

Atypical Hyperplasia

This is a diagnosis that can be made only by a pathologist studying breast tissue removed during a biopsy. Atypical hyperplasia means that there are more cells in a milk duct than there should be and that the cells have some abnormal features. However, the changes seen are definitely not malignant. No one knows what atypical hyperplasia signifies. It may be a threat in and of itself or a sign of some undetectable change elsewhere in the breast. In any case, when atypical hyperplasia is detected, affected women have about three times the normal risk of breast cancer. Those with atypical hyperplasia plus a family history of breast cancer have up to eleven times the normal risk.

THE PREGNANCY EFFECT

The rate of breast cancer is lower than normal among women who were in their twenties when their children were born. (Risks are lowest among women who gave birth to four or more children before the age of thirty.) No one knows why the age at first pregnancy should lower a woman's breast cancer risk, but an intriguing theory holds that breast tissue may be particularly vulnerable to carcinogens during the years between a woman's first menstrual period and her first pregnancy. If so, the sooner pregnancy occurs, the smaller this so-called "window of vulnerability." Some evidence to support this hypothesis comes from observations that Japanese women who were teenagers when the bombs were dropped on Hiroshima and Nagasaki had a much higher than normal rate of breast cancer. This may have been due to the effect of radiation on their vulnerable young breasts. The incidence of breast cancer among mature women who survived the bombings also increased but never reached the levels seen among women who were teenagers at the time.

OBESITY

After menopause, obesity increases your chances of developing breast cancer. (The opposite is true of premenopausal women—risks are higher among those who are thin.) Our high-fat, high-calorie diet may be to blame, but the obesity issue is more complex than the question of what you eat or how much you weigh. Take a look at the major findings in this area:

• Women who develop breast cancer tend to be heavier and taller than women who are not affected. One study showed that risks are highest among women who stand taller than five feet five and weigh more than 154 pounds.

• A 1989 study from Australia showed that women who gain more than twenty-two pounds between the ages of twenty-five and thirty-five are more likely to develop breast cancer than those whose weight does not increase so markedly.

• Researchers at the University of South Florida College of Medicine have found that overweight women who carry their extra pounds in their abdomens have a higher risk of breast cancer than women who are overweight but carry the excess in their hips and thighs. This so-called abdominal obesity is a known risk for gallbladder disease, heart disease, and diabetes, but the Florida study was the first to associate it with breast cancer. If it isn't obvious, you can determine whether the distribution of your weight fits the high-risk pattern by comparing your waist measurement to your hip measurement. Your risk is normal if your waist size is 73 percent or less than your hip measurement. If it is 80 percent or more than your hips, your breast cancer risk is six times as high as normal. Incidentally, the researchers who conducted this study also noted that hormonal abnormalities associated with breast cancer have been found among abdominally obese women. Losing weight restores the hormonal picture to normal.

• Not only does obesity increase the risk of breast cancer, but a study published in the *Annals of Internal Medicine* in January 1992 showed that cancer recurrence was significantly higher among women who are obese (more than 25 percent over the ideal weight for their height). These women had a recurrence rate about 25 percent higher than women who were underweight or normal weight. The heavier the women were at the time of diagnosis the more likely it was that the cancer had spread to the lymph nodes, but even when it had not, the recurrence rate was higher among the obese women.

The higher risk of breast cancer among overweight women may be due to the fact that estrogen is metabolized in body fat. For this reason, heavy women have higher levels of circulating estrogen than thin women. If long-term estrogen exposure increases the risk of breast cancer, then the higher estrogen levels typical of overweight women could explain the link between obesity and breast cancer. The Australian study that found a higher risk of breast cancer among women who gained twenty-two pounds or more between age twenty-five and thirty-five also showed that the heavier a woman was, the more likely she was to have begun menstruating early and stopped later. This lends even more support to the notion that obesity affects a woman's risk of breast cancer by increasing her exposure to estrogen.

HIGH-FAT DIETS

No one knows precisely how diet contributes to breast cancer. However, the rates of certain types of cancer (including breast cancer) are highest in societies where diets are high in fat. Support for this observed link between dietary fat and cancer has come from laboratory studies showing that animals fed high-fat diets develop cancer more often than animals fed low-fat diets. While interesting, these findings cannot be readily applied to humans: millions of women who eat high-fat diets for their entire lives never develop cancer of any kind.

One of the earliest studies suggesting that diet plays a role in breast cancer showed that Japanese women have a very low rate of the disease—as long as they stay in Japan and continue to eat the traditional very low fat diet. When Japanese women immigrate to the United States and adopt our eating habits, their breast cancer rate begins to increase. Today, the incidence of breast cancer among second generation Japanese women is the same as it is for other American women, suggesting that high-fat diets set the stage for cancer relatively early in life. This theory has been bolstered by animal studies showing that laboratory mice fed low-fat diets since birth are less likely to develop the mouse version of breast cancer than those placed on low-fat diets later in life. Laboratory studies also suggest that breast tumors in mice grow faster when the animals are fed polyunsaturated fats; mice fed omega-three fatty acids from fish oils are less likely to develop breast cancer.

Some researchers suspect that calories, not fat, are to blame for the high rate of breast cancer in the United States and western Europe. One theory along these lines holds that high-calorie diets set the stage for cancer by promoting a rapid rate of growth in childhood and adolescence. This would square with observations that in well-nourished Western societies, girls begin to menstruate at a younger age than they do in countries where nutrition is poor. This earlier menstrual pattern means that estrogen and other female hormones begin circulating earlier in life, perhaps explaining the higher breast cancer rate among women in affluent societies.

Given all of the evidence suggesting a link between diet and breast cancer, should we reduce fat or caloric intake to protect ourselves? While it certainly wouldn't hurt (at least we would be thinner), there is no evidence to show that it would do any good. A Harvard School of Public Health study comparing women whose fat intake was about 40 percent of total calories (the amount of fat in the typical American diet) with those who consumed 30 percent of total calories as fat showed no lower incidence of breast cancer among the women whose diets were lower in fat.

Critics of the Harvard study argue that to see a decreased incidence of breast cancer, fat consumption might have to be even lower, perhaps to less than 20 percent of total calories. Obviously, this subject needs further research. The National Institutes of Health is contemplating a massive, long-term study to evaluate the impact of a low-fat diet on the incidence of breast cancer and heart disease, but this effort is still in the planning stage. To get meaningful results a study would have to continue for at least ten years. Even then, the results may not be definitive. If no difference in breast cancer rates shows up, we still would be left with the possibility that the risk posed by high-fat diets develops early in life and cannot be changed in adulthood.

BIRTH CONTROL PILLS

The question of whether the pill can cause breast cancer has been examined repeatedly in the thirty years since it was introduced. Most studies have failed to find any cause and effect, but some experts believe that we're just getting to the point where information becomes meaningful. One recent study from Boston University School of Medicine showed a fourfold increase in breast cancer among a small group of women who took the pill for ten years or more. All had begun to menstruate before the age of thirteen and none had children. We may have more and better information on this subject once the National Cancer Institute completes a study examining the relationship of the pill, diet, and alcohol to breast cancer development. Results are due in 1993.

ALCOHOL

Although women who drink alcohol are at higher risk for breast cancer than teetotalers, findings in this area are confusing. The latest word on the subject came from a 1988 analysis of sixteen reports published since 1982. Most of the studies reviewed found no connection, but, on balance, the analysis by a team of researchers at the Harvard School of Public Health showed that the more alcohol a woman consumes, the higher her risk of breast cancer.

So far, no one has been able to identify any internal mechanism by which alcohol could cause breast cancer. Walter C. Willett, M.D., of the Harvard School of Public Health who headed the most highly regarded study confirming the alcohol–breast cancer link, concluded that it probably never will be possible "to prove beyond any doubt that alcohol causes breast cancer in humans." Still, his team's work shows that the risk is higher among women who drink.

RADIATION

Exposure to radiation can be a factor in the development of breast cancer. The higher rate of breast cancer among Japanese women who survived the bombings of Hiroshima and Nagasaki is a case in point. There also is evidence that women who received x-ray treatments for tuberculosis during the 1930s, 1940s, and early 1950s have higher than normal rates of breast cancer. The incidence is highest among women who were between ten and fourteen at the time of exposure.

Exposure to radiation emitted by mammograms does present a tiny risk: one extra case of breast cancer among every 50,000 women over age fifty who have had mammograms every year for ten years. Clearly, the benefits of detecting breast cancer at an early stage far outweigh this minuscule risk of developing a radiation-induced cancer.

MAMMOGRAMS

Estrogen or no estrogen, we have reached the age when we need mammograms. An annual mammogram is a must if you take estrogen; if not, some doctors now feel that every other year is sufficient (although the American Cancer Society still recommends annual mammograms for all women over fifty).

Mammograms can pick up cancers as small as one fifth of an inch, half the size of the smallest tumor that you or your doctor can feel. While these x-rays do a good job of picking up breast cancer as early as two years before it can be felt as a lump, mammograms are not error proof: even those done at the best facilities by the best-trained technicians and interpreted by the most experienced radiologists are wrong 10 percent of the time. Here's why:

• The lump is in an area that couldn't be seen on the x-ray (usually a part of the breast that cannot be captured between the two plates on the mammography machine).

• The lump was hidden by dense breast tissue (this is more common among premenopausal women whose breasts tend to be dense).

• The lump did not look suspicious to the radiologist.

The error rate can be much higher than 10 percent when facilities do not maintain high standards and personnel are not experienced and well trained. Obviously, an error that falsely assures a woman that she is cancer-free would deprive her of the advantage of early detection. But errors suggesting that cancer is present when, in fact, it isn't also can be financially and emotionally costly. These mistakes will lead to a biopsy and engender enormous heartache and worry. False positive mammograms are extremely common: in the United States nine out of every ten biopsies performed to investigate suspicious mammographic findings are negative (the women do not have cancer).

To reduce your risk of a "false positive" or "false negative" mammogram (and ensure that you are getting the lowest possible dose of radiation) you will have to check out the facilities offering mammograms in your area. The quickest and easiest way to do this is to find out whether the center is certified by the American College of Radiology (ACR). This organization awards certificates to facilities that pass a rigorous inspection and are staffed by well-trained and experienced technicians and radiologists. (You can get a list of certified centers in your state from the ACR. See Appendix 1 for the address and phone number.)

To check out a mammography center for yourself, ask the following questions:

• Is the radiologist who reads the mammograms certified by the American Board of Radiology or the American Osteopathy Board of Radiology?

• If not, has the radiologist had at least two months of full-time training in mammography interpretation, medical radiation physics, radiation effects, and radiation protection?

• How many mammograms does the radiologist interpret or review per year? (Any number above 480 is acceptable.)

• Is the technician certified by the American Registry of Radiological Technologists and/or licensed by the state?

• Do the technicians perform mammograms regularly?

• Is the equipment "dedicated" (designed especially for mammography)?

• Does the mammography machine have a removable grid? (A grid is a device needed to enhance x-ray contrast of the dense breasts typical of premenopausal women.) Since the radiation dose is slightly higher when a grid is used, it should be removed when women whose breasts are not dense are being x-rayed.

• How often is the equipment calibrated? (To ensure that the radiation dose is no more than 0.4 rads per exposure, the equipment should be tested and calibrated at least once a year.)

What's Involved

To get a good x-ray, your breast must be compressed between two flat plates on the mammography machine. Although this can be uncomfortable, it lasts only for the few seconds it takes for the technician to complete positioning you and retreat behind the machine to snap the picture.

When a radiologist is on the premises, he or she probably will look at your mammogram right away to make sure that the picture turned out and see what it shows. Some radiologists come out to tell you that everything is okay. If something suspicious shows up, the radiologist may suggest an ultrasound exam to see if the lump is solid or a cyst. In some centers, this can be done on the spot.

When a radiologist is not available, you will have to wait a few days for your results. If your doctor referred you to the center, the report will go to his or her office and you will have to telephone for your results. If you have a mammogram in a mobile van or center where only mammograms are performed, results are usually mailed to you. These high-volume facilities can provide low-cost mammograms because they are staffed by technicians, not physicians. At the end of the day, all the mammograms go to radiologists for interpretation. Many of these facilities are excellent, but as with any center, check them out first.

BENEFIT VS. RISK

It is important to realize that all the risks described in this chapter don't have the same weight: family history, reproductive history, and menstrual patterns carry the most weight. So, if you have no family history of breast cancer, you had your first child during your twenties, and/or you did not begin to menstruate early or reach menopause late, you probably would not appreciably add to your risk of the disease by taking estrogen if you need it to protect against osteoporosis and heart disease or to overcome hot flashes or other disruptive menopausal symptoms.

If you do have one or more of these risk factors, you might want to consider taking estrogen only for some compelling reason (such as a high risk of osteoporosis or heart disease). If you have a family history of breast cancer and osteoporosis or breast cancer and heart disease, you might want to explore tamoxifen, an option that may afford protection against all three diseases.

TAMOXIFEN

Tamoxifen, a synthetic hormone used to prevent recurrences among women with estrogen-dependent breast cancer, is being studied as a means of preventing breast cancer in healthy women. In 1992 the National Cancer Institute launched a five-year study in which 16,000 women will be given either tamoxifen or a placebo. If tamoxifen proves as effective a preventive measure as some researchers suspect it will, all postmenopausal women may be advised to take it for the rest of their lives!

Tamoxifen prevents estrogen from entering tumor cells by jamming the receptors. Although usually described as an "antiestrogen," the drug acts like estrogen in two important respects: it strengthens bone and appears to protect against heart disease by lowering cholesterol levels.

This isn't as wonderful as it sounds. Because tamoxifen blocks estrogen from entering cells throughout the body, it leads to particularly severe hot flashes and other menopausal symptoms. Some studies have shown that tamoxifen can cause depression, and it also seems to increase the risk of endometrial cancer. Also on the downside: animal studies suggest that tamoxifen may cause liver cancer. So far, no increase in the rate of liver cancer has been seen among the thousands of women who have taken tamoxifen for many years to prevent breast cancer recurrence. However, in 1992 British doctors reported that several women taking tamoxifen developed serious benign liver disease; one died.

We won't know whether tamoxifen can protect healthy women until 1996 when the National Cancer Institute study ends. However, the drug is widely available and some doctors already prescribe it to healthy women at high risk of breast cancer. This approach to the dilemma of how to protect our breasts as well as our bones and hearts is certainly not risk free, but it may be the answer for some women unable or unwilling to take estrogen.

❽ 🅔🅘🅖🅗🅣

A Shock
to the System

DID YOU KNOW that 25 percent of all American women reach menopause on the operating table in the course of a hysterectomy? When the ovaries are surgically removed, as they usually are among women past forty undergoing hysterectomy, the result is instant menopause. With a few flicks of the scalpel, a surgeon forever extinguishes the primary source of estrogen. This is always an enormous shock to the system. The younger a woman is at the time of the operation, the more physically traumatic her estrogen loss will be. If estrogen is not replaced soon after surgery, a woman can expect to develop hot flashes and other menopausal symptoms that will be much more severe than they are when the estrogen supply dwindles gradually as menopause approaches naturally. What's more, without estrogen replacement, a woman's risk of both heart disease and osteoporosis skyrocket.

I got a firsthand account of the impact of this estrogen loss from Glenda Abramson, an outspoken high school classmate who told me she had resisted hysterectomy for years despite fibroids that had gotten so big that she swears she looked pregnant. She had not yet reached menopause when she finally agreed to the operation. "I had my period when I entered the hospital," Glenda recalled. She was totally unprepared for the aftermath of the hysterectomy. "The day after the surgery I went crazy," she reports. "I was so depressed. I was sobbing hysterically. I never knew it was possible to feel that awful. I was screaming for help." Her spirits began to lift a few days later after she began to take estrogen. Now she takes it daily although she worries about the breast cancer risk: "I'm afraid to take it," she told me, "and I'm afraid to stop."

Most women know relatively little about hysterectomy and its aftermath. If they were better informed, perhaps more would refuse the surgery. Few women realize that by agreeing to have their ovaries removed, they are consenting to their own castration. I have always wondered how many would go ahead with the operation if doctors used the word "castration" when recommending the removal of the ovaries. If you think I am overstating the case, look up "castration" in the dictionary. You will see that it means "the removal of the testicles *or the ovaries.*" When a man loses his testicles, he can say goodbye to his sex life. His bones begin to thin, his beard stops growing, his voice rises. Depression descends and mood swings up and down. Castrated men even get hot flashes! Doctors acknowledge that castration is terrible for men and should be considered only in life-or-death situations, but many deny that it has a similar effect on women.

If we didn't know that shutting off a woman's estrogen supply means accelerated bone loss, a higher rate of heart disease, hot flashes, vaginal atrophy, and declining sex drive maybe this attitude would be comprehensible. But we do know what happens. When ovaries are removed during a hysterectomy, estrogen replacement is our only weapon against the inevitable and devastating consequences. So all we can do is take it and hope that life holds no surprises that will rule out the only option we have.

THE HYSTERECTOMY SCANDAL

The rate of hysterectomy in the United States is nothing short of scandalous. It is no secret that even by the most conservative medical standards many of these operations are unnecessary. The hysterectomy rate is twice as high here as it is in Great Britain and five times as high as it is in six other western European countries. What's more, the hysterectomy rate differs markedly from one section of the United States to another. Take a look at the table on page 105. You will see that women in the South have almost twice the rate of

Rates of hysterectomies by age and geographic region, United States: 1965–87

Age and region	1972	1973	1974	1975	1976	1977	1978	1979	1980	1981	1982	1983	1984	1985	1986	1987
						Rate per 1000 population										
15 and over																
United States	8.3	8.7	8.6	8.8	8.1	8.3	7.5	7.3	7.1	7.3	6.9	7.1	6.9	6.9	6.6	6.6
Northeast	6.7	7.0	6.5	6.6	5.9	5.8	5.0	5.3	5.3	4.7	4.7	5.4	4.8	4.3	4.4	4.1
Northwest	7.9	8.8	8.8	9.0	8.6	8.5	8.0	7.3	7.5	7.2	7.1	6.8	6.6	6.6	6.8	6.5
South	9.6	9.6	9.5	9.9	9.6	9.9	9.2	8.9	8.7	8.7	8.5	8.5	8.3	8.3	7.6	7.4
West	8.9	9.3	9.4	9.6	7.7	8.4	6.8	7.1	6.4	7.9	6.6	6.9	7.2	7.8	7.0	8.1
15–44 years																
United States	8.9	9.2	9.1	9.3	8.5	9.1	8.2	8.0	7.6	7.9	7.5	8.0	7.4	7.4	6.9	7.0
Northeast	6.4	6.7	5.8	5.8	5.2	5.3	4.5	4.4	4.9	4.3	4.2	5.0	3.8	3.7	3.6	3.5
Northwest	7.8	8.6	9.3	9.1	8.5	8.7	8.3	7.7	7.7	7.2	7.1	7.5	6.7	6.5	7.0	6.7
South	11.7	11.5	11.2	12.0	11.3	12.0	11.1	11.0	10.3	10.7	10.5	10.8	10.0	9.9	8.9	8.4
West	9.0	9.4	9.3	9.0	7.6	9.3	7.1	7.6	5.9	7.9	6.7	6.9	7.9	8.2	6.8	8.7
45–64 years																
United States	10.0	10.9	10.1	11.0	10.1	9.5	8.7	8.3	8.8	8.3	7.8	7.7	8.1	8.1	8.1	8.0
Northeast	9.3	10.1	9.5	10.2	8.8	8.3	7.2	8.0	7.6	6.9	6.6	7.9	8.4	6.5	7.3	6.2
Northwest	10.8	12.4	10.9	12.4	11.7	10.8	10.1	8.9	9.2	9.5	9.1	8.3	8.7	8.8	8.9	8.5
South	9.0	9.5	10.2	9.1	10.1	9.6	9.2	8.1	8.8	7.5	7.8	7.0	8.0	8.4	7.5	7.9
West	11.5	12.3	12.1	13.7	9.7	9.2	8.1	7.9	9.6	9.7	7.6	8.0	7.0	8.6	9.3	9.7
65 and over																
United States	2.7	2.6	3.3	3.2	3.2	3.2	2.9	3.3	3.1	3.7	3.7	3.2	3.6	3.5	3.3	3.4
Northeast	2.7	1.9	3.3	3.0	3.4	3.1	2.9	3.7	2.9	2.9	3.4	3.0	2.9	3.2	2.7	3.3
Northwest	2.8	3.2	3.4	2.5	3.6	3.6	3.4	3.5	4.5	3.6	4.2	2.6	3.8	4.1	3.3	3.5
South	2.5	2.5	2.4	3.4	2.2	3.1	2.4	2.7	2.2	3.5	3.1	3.0	3.2	2.3	3.2	3.4
West	2.9	3.0	4.7	4.3	4.2	3.2	3.3	3.4	2.9	5.2	4.4	5.1	4.9	5.2	4.1	3.7

Source: National Center on Health Statistics, National Hospital Discharge Survey.

hysterectomies as women in the Northeast. The Midwest comes in second, the West Coast, third. No one has ever come up with a good medical explanation for these discrepancies. There is no evidence that Southern women have a higher rate of gynecological disorders to account for the region's high rate of hysterectomy. The differences between the rate of surgery in the United States, Great Britain, and the rest of Europe also cannot be explained by a higher rate of gynecological disorders among American women. Nor is there any evidence that European women are any less healthy than we are or suffer or die from gynecological disorders because they do not have as many hysterectomies as we do.

UNDERSTANDING HYSTERECTOMY

Technically speaking, hysterectomy means the removal of the uterus. However, the term often is misapplied to take in more extensive surgery in which the fallopian tubes and ovaries also are removed. If only the uterus is involved, the operation is called a "simple" hysterectomy. If the ovaries and tubes are also removed,

Number and Rate of Women Having a Hysterectomy, United States: 1965–87

| | Number | | | Rate | |
| | 1000s | | Percent | Per 1000 Women | |
Year	All Ages	Ages 20–49	Ages 20–49	All Ages	Ages 20–49
1965	426	322	75.6	6.1	8.8
1967	478	371	77.6	6.6	9.9
1969*	508	385	75.8	6.8	9.9
1971	569	434	76.3	7.3	10.8
1973	689	533	77.4	8.5	12.8
1975	724	548	75.7	8.6	12.7
1977	703	542	77.1	8.1	12.0
1979	639	496	77.6	7.1	10.5
1981	674	511	75.8	7.3	10.3
1983	673	525	78.0	7.1	10.2
1985	670	513	76.6	6.9	9.6
1987	653	499	76.4	6.7	9.2

*Data for 1969 as average estimates of 1968 and 1970.

Source: National Hospital Discharge Surveys, 1965 through 1987, National Center for Health Statistics.

Rate of Hysterectomies by Age, United States: 1985–87

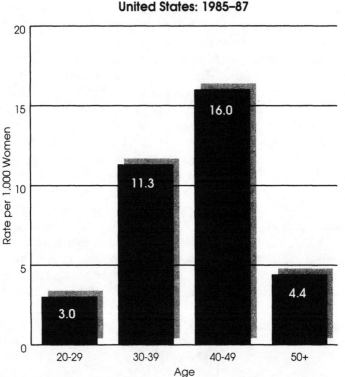

Source: National Hospital Discharge Surveys, 1985–87.

the surgery is termed a "complete" hysterectomy. You may hear the operation described by several other terms:

• *Subtotal hysterectomy:* Removal of the uterus; the ovaries and tubes remain in place.

• *Total hysterectomy:* Removal of the uterus.

• *Total hysterectomy plus tubes and ovaries:* The medical terminology for this operation is hysterectomy with bilateral salpingo-oophorectomy (or ovariectomy).

If only the ovaries are removed (or just one ovary, as sometimes happens when an ovarian cyst or other growth cannot be excised without damaging the ovary itself), the surgery is called oophorectomy or ovariectomy.

Obviously, if you have a hysterectomy, you cannot get pregnant and no longer will menstruate. But if you are premenopausal, as long as you have your ovaries you *should* have plenty of estrogen to protect your bones and your heart. "Should" is the key word in that sentence, because about half of all women who have had "simple" hysterectomies complain of menopausal symptoms that begin soon after the surgery. These discomforts include hot flashes, depression, joint aches and pains, urinary problems, headaches, dizziness, insomnia, and extreme fatigue. The best explanation for this so-called post-hysterectomy syndrome is that the blood supply to the ovaries may be disturbed in the course of the operation, putting them out of the hormone-producing business long before they normally would have shut down. There is also some thought that the post-hysterectomy syndrome stems from the removal of the uterus itself. Although most doctors believe that the uterus serves only one purpose—to nurture a pregnancy—others suspect that it plays a much larger, poorly understood, and largely unrecognized role in women's health. There is some evidence that hormones called prostaglandins produced in the uterus are needed for normal ovarian function. Prostaglandins are also secreted by the cervix and may have unrecognized effects on the nervous system that would disappear if the cervix is removed during hysterectomy. The uterus also appears to produce beta endorphins, secretions that help maintain feelings of emotional well-being.

Sex After Hysterectomy

Certainly, the loss of the uterus can bring on profound sexual changes, although most doctors would dispute this point. A little background on this subject may be useful here. A century ago, medical thinking held that hysterectomy could do wonders to curb a woman's sex drive. It was the treatment of choice for such "perversions" as masturbation and promiscuity. Times have changed. Today, women who complain about loss of sexual feelings after hysterectomy are likely to be told that the ovaries and/or uterus have *nothing* to do with a woman's sexual desire or drive. But that is illinformed nonsense. The discovery by William Masters and Virginia Johnson that the uterus contracts rhythmically during sexual excitement explains why so many women accustomed to this kind of orgasm complain that they are no longer orgasmic after hysterectomy.

Some of the sexual changes may also be related to the removal of the cervix, a structure well equipped with nerve endings that, when stimulated by the thrusting of the penis during intercourse, can produce intensely pleasurable sensations. Cervical mucus also contributes to lubrication during intercourse. Once the cervix is gone, lubrication will be less profuse. In 1979 Pentti P. Kilkku, M.D., a surgeon in Finland, conducted a study to evaluate differences between total (taking it all out) and subtotal (leaving the cervix) hysterectomy. His results showed that after total hysterectomy women were much less likely to experience orgasm than before their operations. The women who had had the subtotal hysterectomies fared much better.

There is also scientific logic to complaints that hysterectomy robs a woman of her sexual interest and drive. If interest in sex wanes after menopause as ovarian hormone levels continue their downward spiral, removing the ovaries will have a similar but more dramatic effect. Since hysterectomy can compromise the normal functioning of ovaries left in place after surgery, the resulting decline in hormone output would correlate with a change in sexual feelings. Doctors who maintain that estrogen replacement helps women maintain active sex lives after menopause can't have it both ways and take the position that the ovaries and the natural hormones they produce have nothing to do with sex drive.

MENOPAUSE AFTER HYSTERECTOMY

Women whose ovaries are left in place after hysterectomy continue to ovulate (the eggs are expelled into the abdominal cavity and absorbed) until hormone production begins to wane as menopause approaches. But since you do not menstruate after a hysterectomy, you don't have the tell-tale menstrual irregularities that usually signal the approach of menopause. Eventually, however, estrogen levels will fall so low that hot flashes or some other symptoms develop. The flashes can come as a big surprise to women who assume that the ovaries as well as the uterus were removed during a hysterectomy.

WHY HYSTERECTOMY?

Most hysterectomies are performed on women between fifteen and forty-four, although about 40 percent of all patients are over forty-five. The table on page 107 will give you a picture of the age breakdown. Hysterectomy is warranted when a woman has cancer of the uterus, ovaries, or vagina; in the case of an obstetrical hemorrhage (a rare, but dangerous event); or when cancer originating elsewhere has spread to the uterus. However, these conditions account for only 9 percent of all hysterectomies. The vast majority of these operations are performed for a variety of benign conditions. Although the symptoms of some of these disorders may be uncomfortable, even intolerable, none are life-threatening and all can be treated in some other way.

Fibroids

Large or troublesome fibroids are the most common indication for hysterectomy. (For a complete discussion of fibroids see Chapter

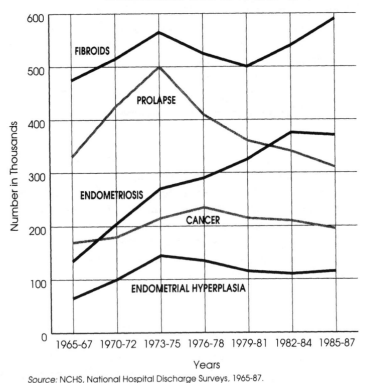

Number of Hysterectomies by Diagnosis and Year, United States: 1965–67 to 1985–87

Source: NCHS, National Hospital Discharge Surveys, 1965-87.

Three.) Although fibroids usually don't cause trouble, a gynecological rule of thumb holds that a hysterectomy can be justified whenever the growths expand the uterus to the size of a twelve-week pregnancy. Doctors have enormous leeway in interpreting this twelve-week rule. Some will eagerly rush in and operate as soon as possible. Others may take a "wait and see" stance—the fibroids may not get bigger. And, since fibroids shrink when estrogen levels drop, a woman nearing menopause usually can opt to wait it out rather than submit to surgery as long as she can tolerate any symptoms her fibroids may be causing.

Hysterectomy is not the only alternative for women with large or troublesome fibroids. An operation called myomectomy in which only the fibroids themselves are removed can usually be substituted. Although this surgery is often reserved for young women who want to preserve their fertility, there is no age limit. However, myomectomy is trickier surgery than hysterectomy, requiring more skill on the part of the surgeon. It also carries a slightly higher risk of hemorrhage. And, there is always the possibility that a woman will develop a new crop of fibroids. For all of these reasons, it can be hard to find a doctor willing to perform a myomectomy on a woman who has completed her family. Most gynecologists subscribe to the view that hysterectomy is more appropriate surgery for any woman who has had all the children she wants. And most will take advantage of the opportunity to remove the ovaries of any woman over forty.

Endometrial Hyperplasia

About 6 percent of all hysterectomies are performed for endometrial hyperplasia. The abnormal bleeding associated with this condition usually occurs among women between the ages of forty-six and fifty-five, the years when we are going through the hormonal upheavals leading to menopause. Endometrial hyperplasia can be detected via an endometrial biopsy performed to investigate the abnormal bleeding. If not treated, the condition can progress through several stages until it becomes "atypical hyperplasia," meaning that the cells are abnormal although not malignant.

In most cases, all stages of endometrial hyperplasia can be eliminated by treatment with progestin. The dose and the length of treatment depend on the stage of the hyperplasia. Unchecked, endometrial hyperplasia can progress to endometrial cancer, which will require a hysterectomy. But should hysterectomy be recommended for any endometrial changes short of cancer, your best bet is to find a doctor willing to treat you with progestin. Since this is standard treatment today, it should not be difficult to locate a gynecologist who will take this approach. Surgery should be considered only in the unlikely event that progestin treatment fails.

Uterine Prolapse

Due to weakening muscular support, the uterus can begin to sag. This happens most often to women who have had a lot of children. If not corrected, the drooping will worsen until the uterus drops into the vagina. In severe cases, it may actually descend through the vagina and protrude from the body. Not surprisingly, a prolapsed uterus can be enormously uncomfortable. What's more, it can weaken the bladder to the point that affected women become incontinent.

Fortunately, a prolapse can often be corrected long before it becomes so serious that surgery must be considered. Exercises to strengthen the weakened muscle supports can help. However, you must begin as soon as the first signs of sagging are detected by your gynecologist in the course of a routine pelvic exam.

The muscle-strengthening exercises to treat prolapse were developed in the 1940s by Arnold Kegel, M.D., as a means of controlling urinary incontinence. All you have to do is work the pubococcygeal muscles that relax when you urinate and contract when you want to stop or prevent the flow of urine. To make sure you are working the right muscles try the exercise while you are urinating. If the flow stops, you are right on target. You can strengthen these muscles by contracting them five times per hour.

Prolapse is the most common reason for hysterectomy among women over the age of fifty-five. When the problem becomes severe enough to warrant surgery, the only alternative to hysterectomy is an operation to resuspend the uterus—that is, to put it back where it was. However, results are not always successful—or permanent—and it may not be easy to find a doctor with the surgical skills needed to perform the operation.

Other Indications for Hysterectomy

Hysterectomies are also performed to treat cervical abnormalities, pelvic infections, endometriosis, and the symptoms of premenstrual syndrome (PMS).

Cervical disorders are most common among women in their twenties and usually are picked up on Pap smears. Short of cancer, most of these abnormalities can be treated and cured with limited surgery although some doctors still recommend hysterectomy if a woman has had all the children she wants.

Pelvic infections also are most common among women in their teens and twenties and usually stem from untreated sexually transmitted diseases. Antibiotics can usually bring these infections under control, but hysterectomy may be recommended as a last resort when stubborn infections persist or infections or the scar tissue they leave behind cause terrible pain.

Endometriosis (see Chapter Three for more on this subject) usually becomes less troublesome as menopause approaches. Hysterectomy may be recommended, but if all the wayward tissue isn't removed, the surgery won't do much good. Nevertheless, endometriosis is second only to fibroids as an indication for hysterectomy.

PMS can be tough to treat, but hysterectomy isn't the answer. Unfortunately, some doctors recommend removing the ovaries, the source of the hormones that appear to underlie the problem. Since affected women are certainly premenopausal, this incomprehensible strategy merely substitutes one set of intolerable problems for another: instead of PMS, a woman will have to contend with menopausal symptoms that will arrive in force as soon as the ovaries are removed. Now, for relief, she will need to replace the estrogen she no longer produces naturally.

WHY SO MANY HYSTERECTOMIES?

In 1977 a committee of the American College of Obstetrics and Gynecology (ACOG) looked into the regional disparities in the rate of hysterectomy in the United States and found no explanation other than "differences in the training of physicians, the style of medical practice and the availability of gynecologists and hospital beds per capita." Nothing has changed since then: no effort to unify thinking among surgeons, no reassessment of the indications for hysterectomy.

But the differences in medical style can't explain everything. There also is the question of attitude toward the uterus on the part of male physicians (and, often, the women doctors men train). Many view it as a nuisance, a "disposable" organ with no function once a woman has had all the children she wants. In 1969 a Connecticut gynecologist named Ralph C. Wright actually proposed in an article in the journal *Obstetrics and Gynecology* that the uterus be removed in every woman past childbearing age. Why? Because "after the last planned pregnancy [it] becomes a useless, bleeding, symptom-producing, potential cancer bearing organ," he argued. His preposterous proposal actually was debated by his colleagues at an ACOG meeting in 1971. Luckily, it went no further.

Still, attitudes toward the uterus and the ovaries remain intransigent: most doctors see no reason to save a uterus if a woman has completed her family and dismiss patients who complain of physical, emotional, and sexual problems after hysterectomy as attention-seeking neurotics.

AND WHAT ABOUT THE OVARIES?

On the face of it, the rationale for removing the ovaries as well as the uterus at hysterectomy seems simple and humane: to protect women from ovarian cancer. This is a terrible disease for which there is no early diagnosis. Because most cases are advanced by the time they are detected, only 20 percent of all victims survive for five years. Eliminating the risk of this disastrous disease might be medically prudent if the trade-off were not so ludicrous. In the first place, ovarian cancer is a relatively rare disease. It develops in only one out of every seventy women. By projecting this incidence across the population, it has been estimated that to save just one woman from the disease, doctors would have to remove ovaries from at least 1500 others!

Given the knowledge that removing a woman's ovaries places her at extremely high risk of both osteoporosis and heart disease, disorders that are responsible for many, many more deaths than ovarian cancer, it is difficult to understand why this practice continues. Does it make sense to deliberately raise a woman's risk of two common killers in order to protect her from a rare one? But, in fact, most surgeons routinely remove the ovaries of all women over forty who are undergoing hysterectomy.

Celso-Ramon Garcia, M.D., director of infertility surgery at the Hospital of the University of Pennsylvania, has been campaigning against this practice for years without a whole lot of success. He maintains that even aging ovaries continue to secrete hormones that

**Percent of Hysterectomies With a Bilateral Oopherectomy,
United States: 1985–87**

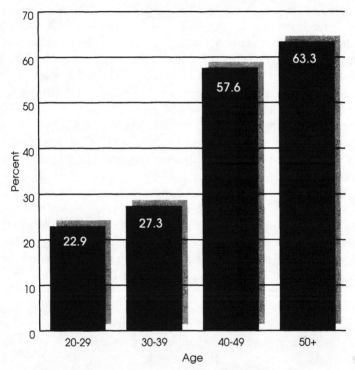

Source: NCHS, National Hospital Discharge Surveys, 1985–87.

may protect against heart disease and osteoporosis. He also argues that the ovaries may act "in other ways not yet scientifically understood to support the well-being and general health of older women." Moreover, he notes that current scientific understanding of maturing ovaries in maintaining the female sex drive is "primitive" at best.

OVARIAN CANCER: THE REAL RISKS

Removing the ovaries at hysterectomy makes sense only if there is something wrong with them or if a woman has a family history of ovarian cancer. More than two affected relatives raise your risk unacceptably high. Steven Piver, M.D., director of the Gilda Radner Familial Ovarian Cancer Registry at the Roswell Park Cancer Center in Buffalo, New York, warns that women with only one affected relative "could be sitting on a time bomb, but we're not sure what their susceptibility is."

Piver recommends that women with two or more affected relatives have their ovaries removed as soon as they have had all the children they want. He is not alone in this seemingly radical view. Henry Lynch, M.D., director of the Hereditary Cancer Institute at Creighton University in Omaha, Nebraska, also advises women at high risk to get rid of their ovaries as soon as their families are complete. However, even this drastic step provides no guarantee. Women from high-risk families who have had their ovaries removed have been known to develop a rare type of abdominal cancer called intra-abdominal carcinomatosis, which is indistinguishable from ovarian cancer.

In addition to family history, the risk of ovarian cancer rises with age and is slightly higher than normal among women who have not had children or were over thirty when their children were born. Infertile women and those with menstrual difficulties such as painful periods and premenstrual tension also have a slightly elevated risk. A high-fat diet also appears to play a role: a 1984 study at Harvard Medical School found that women with ovarian cancer are more likely to use whole milk and butter and less likely to consume skim milk, margarine, and fish than unaffected women. Exposure to asbestos also places women at a higher than normal risk. Particles of asbestos usually found in talcum powder may explain why women who use talc have a slightly higher than normal rate of ovarian cancer.

Women at lowest risk are those who have had multiple pregnancies. Taking birth control pills also significantly lowers the risk even among women who have taken them for as little as three to six months. Some researchers suspect that both multiple pregnancies and the effects of the pill may give the ovaries a needed respite from the stimulation of monthly ovulation.

DETECTING OVARIAN CANCER

Since the risk of ovarian cancer increases with age (average age at diagnosis is fifty-five), a test to detect the disease early would profit everyone. However, at present there is no dependable way to spot ovarian cancer in its earliest curable stages.

An ordinary pelvic exam won't do it because a cancer can be

advanced before the ovary enlarges. Still, it isn't a good idea to neglect this exam. Dr. Piver told me that some tumors the size of grapefruits detected during routine pelvic exams turn out to be curable early stage ovarian cancer. However, since the ovaries shrink after menopause, any enlargement in a postmenopausal woman is cause for concern and must be evaluated promptly. Ovarian enlargements in premenopausal women usually turn out to be harmless cysts.

You definitely cannot depend on a widely publicized blood test for CA-125, an antibody produced by ovarian cancer cells. This test is so unreliable that it may do a woman much more harm than good. In the first place, it misses early tumors as often as it detects them. What's more, it can be "positive" in response to all kinds of conditions that have nothing to do with cancer: normal menstruation, endometriosis, ectopic pregnancy.

The CA-125 test *is* valuable as a means of monitoring a woman who is being treated for ovarian cancer. If levels are normal, treatment can be considered successful. CA-125 levels that are higher than normal usually indicate that the treatment has failed and the cancer has returned.

Unfortunately, the publicity surrounding comedian Gilda Radner's death from ovarian cancer focused the public spotlight on CA-125, and now it is being misused as a test for cancer. Once a test is positive—even though there is a 50 percent chance that it is wrong—you will have to undergo all sorts of diagnostics, including surgery to take a look at your ovaries. In some cases, hysterectomy and removal of the ovaries may be recommended. This could be a lifesaver if cancer is present, but the overwhelming likelihood is that it won't be, and you'll wind up with an operation—and its aftereffects—that you didn't need.

Two other new diagnostic tests being evaluated in combination with CA-125 may prove more useful. One is transvaginal ultrasound, an ultrasound examination of the ovaries conducted via a probe that is inserted in the vagina (this is the same test used to examine the uterus for endometrial hyperplasia as described in Chapter Three). It gives doctors a closer view of the ovaries than ordinary ultrasound (in which the probe is passed over the abdomen) and so far has turned up a number of early cancers. The other new test, transvaginal Doppler color flow imaging, can spot blood vessels that develop to nourish both tumors and benign growths. While all three tests have their limitations, used together they may help detect early stage ovarian cancer.

In the meantime, all we can do if our risks are normal is to get regular checkups. Should hysterectomy be recommended for any reason, weigh the decision carefully. If your surgeon suggests removing the ovaries remember that the younger you are at the time of surgery, the longer you'll have to live without natural estrogen. Even if you are past menopause, don't assume that your ovaries are useless. They probably are still producing some estrogen, and when it comes to the health of your heart and your bones, every little bit helps. Sacrificing your ovaries will protect you from ovarian cancer but keeping them won't raise your risk. It just puts you in the same position as women who haven't had hysterectomies.

If you are having a hysterectomy and decide to hold onto your ovaries, you may have a fight on your hands. Your doctor may disagree with you and refuse to accommodate your decision. Some hospitals have policies *requiring* surgeons to remove the ovaries of all women over forty undergoing hysterectomy. If your doctor is not inclined to respect your wishes, the wisest course of action would be to find another surgeon. Before surgery, you will be asked to give your "informed consent" in writing to the operation. You can specify at the time that your ovaries are to be left in place. But if you give the surgeon the leeway to decide during surgery on the basis of the appearance of the ovaries, you may wake up without them. The best way to hang onto your ovaries is to avoid hysterectomy altogether.

❾ NINE

More Decisions

IF YOU DECIDE to take estrogen, a number of choices await you. Should you take the pill? Or would the patch be better? What about the vaginal cream? Of course, there is always the progestin question. And *how* would you like to take your hormones? Cyclically (three weeks on, one off)? Or continuously, 365 days per year? Undoubtedly your doctor will have strong views on the subject, but you have come this far with the complexities of the estrogen question so you might as well consider the remaining ones. You should also be aware that while estrogen relieves menopausal symptoms among the vast majority of women, it does not always work or may prove effective only at doses considered too high for long-term use.

TESTING, TESTING

Before you get a definite medical go-ahead, you should discuss the subject with your doctor to make sure your thinking jibes. You need to agree on a strategy with which you both can be comfortable. You will also need some medical tests to make sure that you have no health problem or potential problem that could be worsened by estrogen replacement. The tests include:

- A pelvic exam
- A Pap test
- A breast exam
- A blood pressure measurement
- An endometrial biopsy (if you are considering taking estrogen without progestin)
- A mammogram

All this (with the possible exception of the endometrial biopsy) will have to be repeated at least once a year as long as you are taking estrogen.

PILL, PATCH, OR CREAM

The usual way of taking estrogen is in pill form, one tablet per day. This route has two advantages and one big disadvantage. The principal advantage is the protection against heart disease, which appears to be strongest when estrogen is taken orally. Studies have shown that all of the beneficial effects of estrogen on LDL and HDL cholesterol are most pronounced when the hormone is swallowed. The estrogen in the patch lowers LDL but has not been shown to raise HDL. The other advantage to taking estrogen in pill form is that dosage can be more easily adjusted. If you develop symptoms suggesting that you are taking too much or too little estrogen, you can easily take a little more or a little less (under your doctor's supervision) by adding or subtracting pills. The pills are available in a wider range of dosages than other forms of estrogen.

The disadvantage to taking estrogen orally is that to get to the bloodstream it first must pass through the liver. Estrogen's effects on the bile (wastes produced in the liver) can lead to formation of gallstones. Because estrogen can have other unfavorable effects on the liver, women who have problems with impaired liver function cannot take oral estrogen.

The Patch

Estrogen delivered through the patch is absorbed through the skin and goes into the bloodstream without passing through the liver. The actual patch is an adhesive, transparent circle a little larger than a quarter. Estrogen is not the first drug to be administered through the skin. A number of medications, including nitroglycerin needed to relieve angina (chest pain), are "delivered" into the body this way.

The patch is placed on the abdomen or buttocks (*never* the breasts) and must be changed twice a week. Its principal advantage is that the estrogen bypasses the liver. The patch usually is recommended for women who have gallbladder problems or a type of high blood pressure that is affected by angiotensin, an enzyme produced in the liver. The principal disadvantage, as mentioned above, is that the estrogen delivered through the patch does not increase HDL and thus may not have the same protective effect on the heart as oral estrogen. However, the patch is as effective as oral estrogen against bone loss and, in 1991, was approved by the FDA for the prevention and treatment of osteoporosis. The only side effect specific to the patch itself (exclusive of estrogen's side effects) is slight skin irritation that usually can be overcome by moving the patch to a different site. Wearing the patch won't interefere with bathing or swimming—it doesn't come off in the water although it may loosen in humid weather.

Vaginal Creams

Vaginal creams are applied via a plunger similar to those used for tampon insertion. The creams are considered the least effective way of replacing estrogen: while the estrogen supplied does get into the bloodstream and can control hot flashes and other menopausal symptoms, its principal effect is on the vagina and urinary tract.

The main problem with the creams is that there is no way to predict how well they will be absorbed and, therefore, no easy way for doctors to determine the dosage you are getting. Because absorption is so individualized, the creams are not considered effective as protection against osteoporosis. They usually are prescribed only to relieve vaginal dryness or degenerative changes in the urethra. In this area, they can work amazingly fast. Dryness usually disappears within a week, although the estrogen effect may take longer if dryness is severe or if a woman is long past menopause. Some women use the estrogen creams to restore vaginal tissues and then switch to a nonprescription vaginal lubricant. However, without estrogen, tissues will thin out again, and you will need to resume using the cream intermittently. Apart from taking estrogen orally or using a patch this is the only way to overcome dryness and prevent vaginal tissue from permanently thinning.

Another disadvantage to the creams is their messiness: they tend to dribble out of the vagina. You can overcome this problem by applying the cream at bedtime so the estrogen can be absorbed overnight. However, you do have to avoid sexual intercourse until the cream has been absorbed—if the estrogen gets onto the penis, it can be absorbed into a man's bloodstream.

Other Sources

Aside from the pill, patch, and cream the only other way to take estrogen today is via injection. This is both costly and inconvenient. When only pills and creams were available, giving estrogen by injection was the only dependable way of getting it into the bloodstream without going through the liver. (The cream bypasses the liver, but because of uncertainties about absorption, it is not regarded as a dependable way to administer estrogen.)

A number of other delivery systems are in various stages of development. The Schering-Plough Corporation has applied to the FDA for approval of an estrogen gel that you rub into the skin. The advantage here is that the estrogen is more rapidly absorbed into the bloodstream than the estrogen in pills and breaks down more slowly. As a result, you supposedly get a steadier dose of estrogen with more reliable control of hot flashes. The gel (the brand name is Estrogel) also protects against osteoporosis.

Other estrogen alternatives under study include pellets implanted under the skin (this way you can't forget to take the estrogen); a vaginal ring that works on the same sort of absorption principle as the patch; vaginal suppositories; and creams that can be absorbed into the bloodstream after being rubbed on the skin.

SIDE EFFECTS

Estrogen replacement can lead to a number of side effects: water retention, sore or tender breasts, weight gain, nausea, vaginal discharge, headaches, and (rarely) allergic reaction. The water retention is probably responsible, at least in part, for the breast discomfort and weight gain. All three problems are supposed to be temporary and disappear when your body accustoms itself to the renewed supply of estrogen. This should take between two and three months. Sometimes, breast tenderness is due to too high an estrogen dosage. If so, adjusting the dose may eliminate the problem. In severe cases, a small amount of the male hormone testosterone (a form of androgen) may be prescribed or your doctor may switch you to an estrogen-testosterone combination pill.

The vaginal discharge can be a big surprise—it is the result of increased cervical secretions in response to the estrogen. This, too, supposedly can be corrected with an estrogen dosage adjustment. Nausea, said to be the most frequent complaint, often can be overcome by taking estrogen at bedtime, the theory here being that if you are asleep, the nausea won't bother you. Headaches can be more problematical. Adjusting the estrogen dose may help but doesn't always, particularly among women who suffered with "hormonal headaches" during their premenopausal years.

More serious side effects include irregular bleeding (possibly indicating hyperplasia or endometrial cancer), breast lumps, pain or heaviness in the legs or chest (possibly indicating a blood clot), severe headache, dizziness, and changes in vision.

Only one of the women I interviewed mentioned encountering an estrogen side effect. She experienced some breast tenderness but did not consider it bothersome enough to warrant a phone call to her physician. Most of the women I spoke to who were taking estrogen had decided to use it to relieve severe hot flashes or combat vaginal dryness. Perhaps they were so grateful for the relief that they ignored or minimized any side effects. (The woman who reported the breast tenderness had not had any menopausal symptoms—not a single hot flash—and was taking estrogen only because her mother had severe osteoporosis and, like her mother, she is thin and small boned.) When she talked to *Allure* magazine about menopause and estrogen replacement, Jane Fonda said she had gained weight ("a cushion of squishiness") when she began to take estrogen but the extra weight disappeared after six months.

How Much? How Often?

How much estrogen do you need? Enough to do the job—eliminate hot flashes or other menopausal symptoms and, if you consider yourself at risk of osteoporosis, protect your bones. The minimum effective dose for prevention of osteoporosis is 0.625 mg (although, as explained in Chapter Five, 0.3 mg plus 1500 mg of calcium may work, too). However, if you have severe hot flashes you may need a higher dose in the beginning. Doctors usually start women off with 0.625 mg and increase the dosage if hot flashes don't disappear. After symptoms have been under control for a while, the dosage usually can be reduced to 0.625 mg. The goal always is to take the *minimum* effective dose.

The patch comes in two dosages, 0.05 mg, which is equivalent to 0.625 mg of oral estrogen, and 0.10 mg for women who require a higher dose for relief of severe menopausal symptoms.

Vaginal cream comes in doses ranging from 0.01 mg to 1.5 mg.

Whether they use the pill or the patch, most women take estrogen three out of four weeks per month or for twenty-five days per month. The usual routine is to add progestin on days fourteen through twenty-five. However, some doctors recommend taking both estrogen and progestin every day. This strategy is designed to get around the monthly bleeding that occurs when you take estrogen and progestin cyclically. More about that below.

Vaginal creams are prescribed primarily to overcome vaginal dryness. As soon as matters improve, the cream can be used only once every three weeks to keep tissues healthy.

THE PROGESTIN QUESTION

As you know, progestin was added to estrogen replacement to reduce the higher than normal risk of endometrial cancer that occurs when estrogen is taken alone. But, of course, progestin is not trouble free. The most worrisome problem is the potentially increased risk of breast cancer (discussed in Chapter Seven) and the fact that progestin may cancel out some of estrogen's protection against heart disease (see Chapter Six). The extent of these two threats has not yet been fully evaluated, but even before they were recognized, many women objected to taking progestin because it brought back their periods.

Strictly speaking, the bleeding you get when you take progestin isn't a period. Since you are not ovulating, it has no reproductive function. But the combination of estrogen and progestin does mimic the menstrual cycle: estrogen stimulates the endometrium to build up, progestin enters the picture and helps matters along. After progestin is withdrawn (when you stop taking both hormones on day twenty-five), the endometrial buildup is shed. This bleeding is predictable and scheduled. It is engineered not by your normal hormonal cycle but by the cycle you have created by taking estrogen and progestin.

This "withdrawal bleeding" (so called because it occurs upon withdrawal of progestin) is the main reason that women resist estrogen replacement and the primary reason that women who decide to take estrogen change their minds and quit. Although study after study of "compliance" with estrogen replacement therapy show that bleeding discourages women from taking hormones, my own informal survey turned up only one woman who mentioned bleeding as a drawback. She gave up taking estrogen because of "unbelievably heavy" bleeding but later decided she could cope with bleeding better than the hot flashes and depression she experienced when she wasn't taking hormones. She is now back on estrogen and progestin.

If you take estrogen on a long-term basis to protect against osteoporosis, the bleeding eventually stops. However, no one can predict when "eventually" will arrive. One study showed that 60 percent of the women taking estrogen and progestin continued to have "periods" beyond the age of seventy.

One way to eliminate the monthly bleeding is to take estrogen and progestin every day—the "continuous" strategy mentioned above. However, not all doctors are convinced that this is the way to go for three reasons: (1) uncertainties about the impact of the unavoidably higher dose of progestin on the protection against heart disease; (2) concerns that the progestin dose is higher than needed to protect the endometrium; and (3) the lack of studies showing any advantage to this strategy other than the absence of periods.

Women who opt for the continuous approach may have some bleeding at first. It may take up to a year of tinkering with dosages to get this system running smoothly, but once it is the "periods" disappear for good.

Dosages

With the cyclical approach the progestin dosage usually is 5 mg for twelve days or 10 mg for ten days. Some doctors will reduce the dosage when women complain of PMS-type symptoms. And, sometimes the dosage must be adjusted to make sure that progestin effectively combats the endometrial cancer risk.

If you take estrogen and progestin every day, the usual dose is 2.5 mg.

PMS? At This Age?

Along with periods, progestin can also bring on such premenstrual symptoms as breast tenderness, fluid retention, weight gain, and depression. This is another reason that women don't like progestin.

The premenstrual symptoms occur in an estimated 5 to 10 percent of all women and rank second to bleeding as the reason women quit taking hormones. In my personal, informal, and very unscientific survey I did not find one woman who complained about this problem, but in her book, *The Silent Passage,* writer Gail Sheehy told a cautionary tale of what progestin did to her:

"It brought on unbelievable physical and emotional symptoms that I'd never experienced before. After a year of the combined hormones, my body seemed to be at war with itself for half of every month. My energy was flagging, and resistance to minor infections was falling. It felt as if I were racing my motor." Sheehy wrote that she felt so horrible that she quit taking hormones "cold turkey." Within two months her hot flashes came back in full force. So she went back to the hormones and found that the progestin effect was even worse than she remembered: "I felt by afternoon as if I had a terrible hangover. . . . It only worsened as the day went on bringing with it a racing heart, irritability, waves of sadness and difficulty concentrating . . . to top it off, the hot flushes came back."

Sheehy's symptoms didn't ring any bells with the women I talked to. Doctors acknowledge that premenstrual symptoms are a big problem for some women taking progestin, but reactions as dramatic as Sheehy's appear to be rare.

ESTROGEN ALONE?

About half the women taking estrogen for postmenopausal symptoms or to prevent osteoporosis do not take progestin. There are four possible reasons: (1) their doctors are behind the times and haven't caught on to the fact that progestin reduces the risk of endometrial cancer; (2) the women don't want to take it because of the bleeding or the PMS; (3) the women have had hysterectomies and don't need it; or (4) questions about progestin's negative effects on the risks of breast cancer and heart disease have convinced their doctors that progestin may do more harm than good.

The fact is that no form of progestin has been approved by the FDA for hormone replacement in postmenopausal women. Furthermore, there have been no long-term studies of progestin's effects beyond its protection against endometrial cancer.

Taking estrogen without the progestin will raise your risk of endometrial cancer. On the other hand, it may reduce any added risk of breast cancer posed by taking progestin. At worst, the risk of endometrial cancer is eight times as high among women taking estrogen alone as it is among those taking no hormones at all. That works out to eight cases per thousand women per year. As for breast cancer, the normal risk for a woman in her early fifties is one in 49, one in 23 for women in their sixties. Since we don't yet know how much (if any) of an additional risk progestin poses, we can't calculate how much it could be reduced by doing without. If it is four times as high, as the Swedish study described in Chapter Seven suggests, the cancer rate for women in their fifties taking both hormones would be four per 49 women; for those in their sixties the risk would be four per 23 women.

But it is important to realize that numbers alone do not tell the full story. While the risk of endometrial cancer is definitely higher than the risk of breast cancer, the disease itself poses a lesser threat.

Endometrial cancer is usually diagnosed in its early stages when it is curable. What's more, the death rate from this disease has declined by 69 percent since 1958. All told the disease appears to present much less of a risk than breast cancer.

In general, breast cancer is a far more serious disease than endometrial cancer even when breast cancer is detected "early." Despite improvements in diagnostics and treatment, the survival rate has not improved during the last few decades. However, there is some evidence from Sweden that breast cancer survival rates are higher than normal among women who develop the disease while taking estrogen than they are among victims who never took hormones. The reasons for the difference have not yet been explained.

As far as heart disease is concerned, there is that nagging possibility that progestin will cancel out estrogen's protective effect. We won't know for sure until results of the PEPI study described in Chapter Six become available. But since we can lower our risks of heart disease by losing weight, exercising, giving up cigarettes if we smoke, and, if necessary, getting treatment for high blood pressure and/or high cholesterol, calculating any increased risk progestin may pose is less urgent at this time.

Hedging Your Bets

If you decide to take estrogen without progestin, your doctor may insist on an annual endometrial biopsy to make sure no suspicious changes are taking place. This biopsy can be done in the doctor's office. It requires insertion of an instrument into the uterus via the vagina to remove a sampling of cells for examination by a pathologist. The procedure can be uncomfortable, but it is certainly cheaper and more convenient than a D & C, which must be done in the hospital under general anesthesia. As an alternative to the endometrial biopsy some doctors now perform a "transvaginal ultrasound," an ultrasound examination of the endometrium in which a probe through which sound waves are passed is inserted in the vagina. The sound waves bounce off the endometrium creating a black-and-white television image that can reveal whether the endometrium has thickened in response to estrogen.

To avoid these annual examinations some doctors recommend taking progestin every three months to prompt the shedding of any estrogen-stimulated endometrial buildup. If nothing happens, the endometrium no longer is responding to estrogen stimulation and you can stop worrying about the increased cancer risk.

WHAT'S THE RUSH?

I, for one, would feel a lot more comfortable about taking estrogen if we knew more about the risks it poses, specifically, the breast cancer risk. Having completed my personal crash course on estrogen replacement I have decided that I don't have to make up my mind immediately. If I develop horrendous menopausal symptoms, I'll probably cross my fingers and ask my gynecologist for a prescription to get me through the worst part. Otherwise, I'm going to wait and see. I don't think my bones will fall apart overnight.

It isn't likely that researchers will have the definitive answers we all want anytime soon. But within the next few years we should know a little more than we do today about the breast cancer risk. I am not willing to add to my personal risks, at least not now. The next few years also may bring a breakthrough on the osteoporosis front that will enable us to protect our bones without risking our breasts. Or maybe future studies will prove more reassuring about the extent of the breast cancer risk posed by estrogen and progestin. And there always is the possibility that researchers will find a better way to protect the endometrium, perhaps some method of delivering progestin directly to the uterus so that it cannot endanger the breasts. As far as heart disease is concerned, so many other strategies are available to reduce our risks that I, for one, would not take estrogen solely to protect my heart (but then I have no family history of heart disease and no personal risk factors).

And if I were you?

I would take estrogen if I had a high risk of osteoporosis and a normal risk of breast cancer.

I would take it if I considered my risk of heart disease high and my risk of breast cancer normal.

I would take it to eliminate intolerable menopausal symptoms.

I would use the vaginal creams to overcome vaginal dryness.

I would NOT take estrogen if my risk of osteoporosis and heart disease is low EXCEPT for the few months or years it may take to relieve severe menopausal symptoms.

I don't expect that there ever will be a risk-free way to protect our bones and hearts and reverse the effects of estrogen deprivation on the vagina. I wish I could be more sanguine about the breast cancer risk we are faced with today when we contemplate estrogen replacement. No woman who develops breast cancer while taking estrogen will ever know that the estrogen was responsible and no woman who avoids estrogen should assume for a moment that she can't get breast cancer. But now that the issue has been raised we all have to deal with it as best we can and hedge our bets so that we are comfortable with the odds. Were it not for my own worries about breast cancer I would happily take any of the other risks estrogen replacement presents.

Instead, I am going to wait and see what comes next. If I can't find a better way to protect my bones during my first year or two past menopause, I probably will take estrogen. Temporarily. Until something better comes along.

QUESTIONS TO ASK YOUR DOCTOR

The questions below assume you have finished reading this book and are now familiar with the benefits and risks of estrogen replacement. If you decide you are going to take it at menopause, you need to talk to your doctor to make sure that you are in agreement about your personal risks and that your thinking jibes.

1. *I haven't had a period for three months. Have I reached menopause?*

Maybe, but you could be pregnant.

2. *How do you evaluate my risks of osteoporosis, heart disease, and breast cancer?*

Your physician will need to take a thorough history. Don't go against your gut instincts if a doctor minimizes what you perceive to be a serious risk.

3. *If I decide to take estrogen replacement, when should I start?*

There are no hard-and-fast rules here. Some doctors will insist on an FSH test to confirm that you are menopausal. Others may write a prescription sooner if you have horrible hot flashes, insomnia, or intolerable vaginal dryness. If you are at high risk of osteoporosis, some experts believe that the sooner you get on estrogen the better. If you do take estrogen before you are absolutely sure you have reached menopause, you need to be followed very carefully to be sure no adverse endometrial changes occur.

4. *Will you prescribe estrogen without progestin?*

No problem if you have had a hysterectomy. If not, some doctors will balk. Taking estrogen alone avoids the return of your "period" and the potentially negative effects of progestin. If you would rather not take progestin, it should not be too hard to find a doctor who agrees with you. On the other hand, if your doctor doesn't prescribe it, and you don't feel comfortable taking estrogen alone, you should switch to a doctor whose approach squares with your wishes.

5. *If I do take estrogen without progestin, will I need an annual endometrial biopsy?*

Some doctors will insist upon this or a transvaginal ultrasound exam to make sure the endometrium is healthy. Others may require an annual check only if you are at high risk of endometrial cancer. Still others may let two or even three years pass between the tests. If your doctor doesn't do any checking, ask why and be sure you feel comfortable with the answer.

CHECKLIST OF ESTROGEN ISSUES

Here is a list of health issues to discuss with your doctor if you are considering estrogen replacement:
1. *Osteoporosis risk*
• Family history
• Race (risk is highest among white women)
• Body build
• Weight

- Amount of exercise you typically get
- Smoking
- Typical calcium intake
- Typical alcohol intake

2. *Heart disease risk*
- Weight
- Weight distribution (abdominal obesity increases your risk)
- Cholesterol level
- Blood pressure
- Physical activity
- Family history
- Smoking

3. *Breast cancer risk*
- Family history
- Tamoxifen (as alternative to estrogen replacement for women at high risk of breast cancer)

4. *Uterine fibroids*
5. *Endometriosis*
6. *Gallbladder disease*
7. *Severity of menopausal symptoms*

APPENDIX 1

Resources

Cancer

The following organizations can provide information on breast and endometrial cancer:

> *American Cancer Society* (ACS)
> 1599 Clifton Road, NE
> Atlanta, GA 30329
> 1 (800) ACS-2345

Or, contact your local division.

The American Cancer Society publishes a wide range of materials about cancer prevention and treatment. All are available free of charge.

Local ACS chapters can provide referrals for mammography.

> *National Cancer Institute* (NCI)
> Building 21/Room 10A 24
> Bethesda, MD 20892
> 1 (800) 4-CANCER

NCI publishes a wide range of materials on cancer prevention and treatment. All are available free of charge. Some are available in Spanish.

American College of Radiology (ACR)
1891 Preston White Drive
Reston, VA 22091
(703) 648-8910

Accredits mammography facilities nationwide. For a list of accredited facilities in your area write to the ACR or telephone 1 (800) 4-CANCER.

Hereditary Cancer Institute
Creighton University
P.O. Box 3266
Omaha, NE 68103-9990
1 (800) 648-8133
(402) 280-2942

Evaluates families to identify hereditary cancer, identifies high-risk relatives in cancer-prone families, provides recommendations for surveillance or early detection check-ups for family members at high risk for cancer, publishes informational materials for families and physicians.

Hysterectomy

Hysterectomy Education and Resource Services (HERS)
422 Bryn Mawr Avenue
Bala Cynwyd, PA 19004
(215) 667-7757

Telephone counseling for women who have been advised to have hysterectomies or who already have had the surgery. Publishes a newsletter and provides information on hysterectomy and available alternatives.

Menopause

A Friend Indeed
Box 1710
Champlain, NY 12919-1710
(514) 843-5730
FAX (514) 843-5681

Publishes a monthly newsletter about menopause, the latest research on the subject, and health topics of concern to women.

Osteoporosis

National Osteoporosis Foundation
2100 "M" Street, NW
Suite 602
Washington, DC 20037
(202) 223-2237

Publishes patient education materials on the prevention and treatment of osteoporosis.

National Institute of Arthritis, Diabetes, Digestive and Kidney Diseases
Building 31/Room 9A04
Bethesda, MD 20205
(301) 496-5877

Publishes patient information on the prevention and treatment of osteoporosis.

Heart Disease

American Heart Association
7320 Greenville Avenue
Dallas, TX 75321
(214) 373-6300

Publishes a wide variety of materials on heart disease treatment and prevention including information on diet, exercise, blood pressure, and cholesterol control.

National Cholesterol Education Program Information Center
4733 Bethesda Avenue
Suite 530
Bethesda, MD 28014
(301) 951-3260

Materials on lowering heart disease risk by reducing cholesterol through diet, exercise, and medical treatment.

Gynecology

The American College of Obstetrics and Gynecology
404 12th Street, SW
Washington, DC 20024-2188

Patient education materials on a wide range of women's health topics including estrogen replacement, menopause, and endometrial cancer. Please make requests in writing and enclose a business-size stamped, self-addressed envelope.

APPENDIX 2

Estrogens and Progestins Used for Hormone Therapy

Brand name	Generic name	Manufacturer
Estrogens		
Estinyl	Ethinyl estradiol	Schering
Estrace	Micronized estradiol	Mead Johnson Labo
Estraderm	Transdermal 17-estradiol	CIBA
Estratab	Esterified estrogen	Reid-Rowell
Estratest	Esterified estrogen with methyl-testosterone	Reid-Rowell
Estratest H.S.	Half-strength Estratest	Reid-Rowell
Estrovis	Quinestrol	Parke-Davis
Menrium	Esterified estrogen plus chlordiazepoxide (anti-anxiety drug)	Hoffman-La Roche
Ogen	Estropipate	Abbott Laboratories
Premarin	Conjugated equine estrogens	Wyeth-Ayerst
Premarin with methyltestosterone	Conjugated equine estrogens plus methyltestosterone	Wyeth-Ayerst
PMB-200, PMB-400	Premarin plus meprobomate (tranquilizing agent)	Wyeth-Ayerst
TACE	Chlororianisene	Marion Merrell Dow
Diethylstilbestrol	DES, synthetic estrogen	Eli Lilly
Menest	Esterified estrogen	SmithKline Beecham
Feminone	Esterified estrogen	Upjohn
Progestins		
Provera	Medroxyprogesterone acetate	Upjohn
Amen	Medroxyprogesterone acetate	Carnick Laboratories
Curretab	Norethindrone acetate	Reid-Rowell
Aygestin	Norethindrone acetate	Wyeth-Ayerst
Norlulate	Norethindrone acetate	Parke-Davis
Norlutin	Norethindrone	Parke-Davis

Source: U.S. Office of Technology Assessment, 1992.

● ● ●

Glossary

Adenocarcinoma: The most common kind of cancer of the uterus.

Adenomatous hyperplasia: Changes in the lining of the uterus usually due to proliferation of cells in response to estrogen stimulation; may indicate a risk of endometrial cancer. Also see *Endometrium; Hyperplasia.*

Adrenals: Glands situated atop the kidneys that secrete a number of hormones including adrenaline, androgen, estrogen, and progestogen.

Aerobic: With air. Often used to refer to exercise that improves the body's use of oxygen.

Amenorrhea: Absence of menstruation.

Androgen: Male sex hormones. Both men and women produce androgen although men produce much more.

Androstenedione: A form of androgen secreted by menopausal ovaries; the major source of estrogen in menopausal women.

Angiotensin: A liver enzyme that may precipitate high blood pressure.

Anovulatory: Absence of ovulation.

Atherosclerosis: Disease that limits the flow of blood through inner walls of arteries. Results from buildup of plaque, a substance composed of fat and cholesterol.

Atrophic vaginitis: The shrinkage of vaginal tissues that occurs after menopause; can cause great discomfort during sexual intercourse.

Atrophy: To wither or degenerate.

Atypical hyperplasia: Precancerous changes in the lining of the uterus or endometrium.

Bellergal: Drug sometimes prescribed for relief of hot flashes; contains phenobarbital and ergotamine.

Benign breast disease: A noncancerous condition. Also see *Fibrocystic breast disease.*

Beta endorphins: Internally produced substances that have a calming effect on the nervous system.

Bilateral salpingo-oophorectomy: Removal of both fallopian tubes and ovaries, usually in the course of a hysterectomy.

Biopsy: Removal of a tissue sample for laboratory studies.

Bisphosphonate: A drug that prevents bone loss by blocking the activity of cells that remove bone tissue.

Black cohosh: An herb sometimes used for relief of hot flashes.

Bladder: The sac that contains urine.

Blood clot: Jellylike mass of blood. Can cut off blood flow to the heart if it lodges in coronary artery.

Blood lipids: Fats or fatty substances in the blood.

Bone densitometry: Medical test to detect bone density.

Bone mass: Total amount of bone tissue.

Breakthrough bleeding: Abnormal uterine bleeding among women on hormone replacement therapy after menopause.

Calcitonin: A hormone used to slow bone breakdown among women with osteoporosis; it is administered by injection.

Calcitriol: A vitamin D compound that prevents bone loss and may help rebuild bone.

Calcium: The mineral needed to maintain bone strength.

Cardiac: Pertaining to the heart.

Castration: Removal of the ovaries or testicles.

Cervix: The entrance to the uterus.

Cholesterol: Substance produced in the body and contained in foods from animal sources, primarily egg yolks, dairy products, and red meat.

Chronic: Of long duration.

Climacteric: The female transition from reproductive to nonreproductive status; begins about ten years prior to menopause and continues for about ten years afterward.

Clitoris: A sexually responsive female genital structure.

Clonidine: A drug for high blood pressure sometimes used to relieve hot flashes.

Collagen: Protein essential to the support of bone, skin, connective tissue, and cartilage.

Combined hormone replacement therapy: Daily doses of estrogen and progestin; as opposed to cyclical hormone replacement therapy. See *Cyclical hormone replacement therapy.*

Compression fracture: Spinal fractures that occur when weakened vertebrae are crushed by body weight.

Coronary arteries: Arteries that supply blood to the heart.

Coronary heart disease: Damage to the heart resulting from reduced blood supply due to narrowing in coronary arteries.

Corpus luteum: Ruptured follicle that once contained an egg; literal meaning is "yellow body" in reference to its yellow color. It secretes both estrogen and progesterone.

Cortical bone: The dense, compact layer that forms the outer portion of bones.

Creatinine: A substance in urine that can be measured as an approximation of calcium excretion.

Cyclical hormone replacement therapy: Hormone replacement administered for twenty-five days per month; estrogen is taken for twenty-five days with progestin from days twelve or fourteen through twenty-five.

Cystic hyperplasia: Cell changes in the lining of the uterus; the least serious of three types of hyperplasia that may precede development of endometrial cancer.

Cystocele: Protrusion of the bladder into the vagina.

D & C: See *Dilatation and Curettage.*

Dilatation and Curettage (D & C): A surgical procedure that involves dilating or widening the cervix and then scraping the endometrium or lining of the uterus with a spoon-shaped instrument called a curette; performed to investigate abnormal uterine bleeding and rule out endometrial cancer.

Double blind study: A study in which neither the participants nor the researcher knows whether any individual taking part is getting the drug or other treatment being tested or a placebo.

Dowager's hump: Upper back deformity due to vertebral fractures characteristic of osteoporosis.

Dual energy x-ray absorptiometry: A technique to measure the amount of bone tissue in the hip and spine.

Dual photon absorptiometry: A means of measuring total cortical and trabecular mineral content of the hip and spine. Also see *Cortical bone; Trabecular bone.*

Dysmenorrhea: Painful menstruation.

Edema: Swelling due to fluid retention.

Endometrium: Lining of the uterus.

Endometrial biopsy: Removal of a tissue sample from the endometrium to examine cells for evidence of disease.

Endometrial hyperplasia: Overgrowth of cells in the lining of the uterus (endometrium) in response to estrogen stimulation; if unchecked, could lead to endometrial cancer.

ERT: See *Estrogen replacement therapy.*

Estraderm: Brand name of transdermal patch used to deliver estrogen through the skin.

Estradiol: The strongest form of estrogen.

Estriol: The weakest natural estrogen.

Estrogen: Primary female sex hormone; produced by the ovaries.

Estrogen replacement therapy (ERT): Treatment to partially replace estrogen after menopause.

Estrone: A weak form of estrogen.

Etridronate: A drug used to treat osteoporosis.

Fallopian tubes: Tubes running from the uterus to the ovaries; sperm and egg meet and mate in the tubes.

Fibrocystic breast disease: A benign breast condition characterized by lumpiness and tenderness.

Fibroid: Benign uterine growth. Also called myoma, leiomyoma.

Follicle: The sac in which eggs develop.

Follicle stimulating hormone (FSH): Hormone released by the pituitary to stimulate maturation of follicles in the ovaries; FSH levels rise as menopause approaches.

Formation: The process by which new bone is made.

Formication: Sensation of insects crawling on the skin; a rare symptom of menopause.

FSH: See *Follicle stimulating hormone.*

Ginseng: An herb of the *Panax* family sometimes used for relief of hot flashes.

Gonadotropin releasing hormone (GnRH): A hormone released by the hypothalamus that instructs the pituitary to release follicle stimulating hormone (FSH) and luteinizing hormone (LH) at different stages of the menstrual cycle.

GnRH: See *Gonadotropin releasing hormone.*

Growth hormone (GH): A hormone that stimulates production of bone-forming cells; it may prove useful in osteoporosis treatment.

HDL: See *High density lipoproteins.*

Heart attack: Damage due to insufficient blood supply to the heart.

High density lipoproteins (HDL): "Good" cholesterol that helps clear deposits of cholesterol away from surfaces where it can stick to and damage artery walls.

Hormones: Body chemicals that stimulate specific physical effects in the body.

Hormone replacement therapy (HRT): Treatment after menopause to partially replace the hormones estrogen and progesterone.

Hot flashes: Waves of heat that can occur intermittently as symptoms of estrogen deprivation; sometimes used to refer to aura or premonition that precedes actual heat wave.

Hot flush: Term sometimes used to refer to hot flash; preferred term in Great Britain.

HRT: See *Hormone replacement therapy.*

Hyperplasia: Proliferation of cells in the endometrium (lining of the uterus) in response to stimulation by estrogen. Also see *Atypical hyperplasia, Adenomatous hyperplasia, Cystic hyperplasia.*

Hypertension: High blood pressure.

Hypothalamus: The brain's control center; located above the pituitary gland.

Hysterectomy: Removal of the uterus.

Hysteroscopy: A surgical procedure in which a thin, light-transmitting viewing scope is inserted into the uerus via the vagina to examine the uterus.

Incontinence: Inability to control urination.

Insomnia: Sleeplessness; a frequent symptom of menopause.

International unit (IU): Standard of measurement applied to hormone level concentrations, some vitamin dosages.

Ischemia: Decreased blood flow, usually due to narrowed or blocked arteries.

Kegel exercises: Exercises designed to strengthen muscles that control urination; sometimes recommended as treatment for urinary incontinence or to prevent mild uterine prolapse from worsening.

Kyphosis: Curvature of spine resulting from fractured vertebrae due to osteoporosis; commonly referred to as "dowager's hump."

Laparoscope: A long, thin surgical device used for examining the pelvic cavity.

LDL: See *Low density lipoprotein.*

Leiomyoma: See *Fibroid.*

LH: See *Luteinizing hormone.*

Libido: Sex drive.

Low density lipoprotein (LDL): A form of cholesterol that contributes to deposits of fat and other material that clog arteries, leading to coronary artery disease and heart attacks. Also see *High density lipoproteins.*

Lupron: A hormonal drug sometimes used to shrink uterine fibroids prior to surgery. Also see *Fibroid.*

Luteinizing hormone (LH): The hormone responsible for rupturing follicles to release eggs for conception.

Mammogram: Breast x-ray.

Menarche: Onset of menstruation.

Menopause: Last menstrual period.

Myoma: See *Fibroid.*

Myoma coagulation: An experimental technique to shrink fibroids (myoma).

Night sweats: Excessive heat and sweating that occur during the night; a symptom of menopause that may be the nighttime version of hot flashes.

Obesity: Excess body fat; increases risk of heart disease, breast cancer.

Oophorectomy: Removal of the ovaries.

Osteoarthritis: The most common form of arthritis; stems from wear and tear on the joints; develops in everyone eventually.

Osteoblast: A cell that helps form bone tissue.

Osteoclast: A cell that resorbs and removes old bone.

Osteoporosis: Disease characterized by thinning of bone.

Ovaries: Female organs responsible for production of eggs, estrogen, and other hormones.

Ovulation: Release of egg from ovaries; occurs on a monthly cycle for most of the premenopausal years.

Oxalates: Compounds found in some leafy green vegetables that interfere with calcium absorption.

Patch: A round adhesive device that delivers estrogen when attached to the skin.

Peak bone mass: Maximum bone strength and density; occurs at about age thirty-five.

Perimenopause: Years immediately preceding menopause.

Phlebitis: Inflammation of a vein due to formation of a blood clot.

Photon: A unit of magnetic energy, which bone and soft tissue absorb at different rates; used in measurement of bone density.

Phytates: Compounds found in grains that can interfere with calcium absorption.

Pituitary: Endocrine gland that orchestrates hormonal activity.

Plaque: Deposits of cholesterol, other fatty substances, and debris in lining of artery walls; can impede blood flow to the heart.

PMS: Premenstrual syndrome; constellation of symptoms that precede menstruation; may worsen as menopause approaches.

Postmenopause: Following menopause.

Premarin: Brand name of the most frequently prescribed estrogen for use by postmenopausal women.

Premenopause: Prior to menopause.

Progestagen: Alternate form of reference to progestin. See *Progestin.*

Progesterone: A hormone produced by the ovaries that interacts with estrogen to control the menstrual cycle.

Progestin: Drug that mimics the effects of progesterone.

Prolapse: Sagging of the uterus, bladder, or vagina due to loss of muscle and ligament support.

Provera: Brand name of a frequently prescribed progestin. See *Progestin.*

Puberty: The period during which an individual becomes capable of reproduction.

Quantitative computed tomography (QCT): A computerized analysis of pinpoint x-rays that provides a measurement of bone density in the spine.

RDA: Recommended dietary allowance for vitamins and minerals.

Resorption: The process during which old bone is dissolved and eliminated.

Salmon-calcitonin: Drug used to slow bone loss among patients with osteoporosis.

Salpingo-oophorectomy: Removal of the ovaries and fallopian tubes.

Single photon absorptiometry: A means of measuring bone mineral content of the forearm, wrist, heel; primarily measures cortical bone. See *Cortical bone.*

Sodium fluoride: Drug used to treat osteoporosis.

Stress: Physical or emotional strain or pressure.

Stress incontinence: Inability to retain urine when laughing, coughing, or exercising.

Subcutaneous: Under the skin.

Subtotal hysterectomy: Surgical removal of the uterus.

Syndrome: A collection of symptoms.

Testosterone: The hormone produced by the testes and in small amounts by the ovaries.

Thiazide diuretics: Drugs used to control high blood pressure, which may help prevent bone loss.

Thromboembolism: A blood vessel blocked by a blood clot.

Thrombophlebitis: See *Phlebitis.*

Total hysterectomy: Surgical removal of the uterus and cervix.

Trabecular bone: The porous, honeycombed interior of bone.

Transdermal: Pertains to medication administered through the skin by means of an adhesive patch.

Triglyceride: Fat in the bloodstream derived from fat in food.

Urethra: A tube that empties urine from the bladder.

Uterus: The female organ; the womb.

Vagina: Muscular canal that extends from the uterus to the exterior of a woman's body.

Vasomotor: Medical term used to describe menopausal symptoms such as hot flashes characterized by dilation of blood vessels.

Vertebrae: The thirty-three bones of the spinal column.

Vitamin D: A nutrient needed for calcium absorption.

Vitamin E: Nutrient derived from oils and whole grains; supplements may relieve hot flashes.

VLDL: Very low density lipoprotein; a form of cholesterol.

Withdrawal bleeding: Uterine bleeding that occurs among postmenopausal women taking estrogen and progestin in a cyclical pattern.

Womb. See *Uterus.*

Bibliography

Breast Cancer

Breast Cancer and Ovarian Cancer: Beating the Odds, Margaret Kemeny, M.D., and Paula Dranov, Addison-Wesley, Reading, MA, 1992.

Dr. Susan Love's Breast Book, Susan M. Love, M.D., with Karen Lindsey, Addison-Wesley, Reading, MA, 1990.

Hysterectomy

Hysterectomy, Before and After, Winnifred B. Cutler, Ph.D., Perennial Library, HarperCollins Publishers, New York, 1990.

How to Avoid Hysterectomy, Lynn Payer, Pantheon, New York, 1988.

Menopause and Hormone Therapy

Women and the Crisis in Sex Hormones, Barbara Seaman and Gideon Seaman, M.D., Bantam Books, New York, 1979.

Menopause: A Guide for Women and the Men Who Love Them, Winnifred B. Cutler, Ph.D., and Celso-Ramon Garcia, M.D., W. W. Norton, New York, 1992.

The Menopause, Hormone Therapy and Women's Health, U.S. Congress, Office of Technology Assessment, U.S. Government Printing Office, Washington, DC, May 1992.

Managing Your Menopause, Wulf H. Utian, M.D., Ph.D., and Ruth S. Jacobwitz, Prentice-Hall Press, New York, 1990.

•••

INDEX